1,000,000 Books

are available to read at

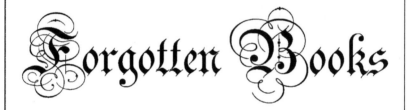

---◆---

www.ForgottenBooks.com

---◆---

Read online
Download PDF
Purchase in print

ISBN 978-1-5284-0198-2
PIBN 10163675

This book is a reproduction of an important historical work. Forgotten Books uses
state-of-the-art technology to digitally reconstruct the work, preserving the original format
whilst repairing imperfections present in the aged copy. In rare cases, an imperfection in
the original, such as a blemish or missing page, may be replicated in our edition. We do,
however, repair the vast majority of imperfections successfully; any imperfections that
remain are intentionally left to preserve the state of such historical works.

Forgotten Books is a registered trademark of FB &c Ltd.
Copyright © 2018 FB &c Ltd.
FB &c Ltd, Dalton House, 60 Windsor Avenue, London, SW19 2RR.
Company number 08720141. Registered in England and Wales.

For support please visit www.forgottenbooks.com

1 MONTH OF
FREE
READING

at

www.ForgottenBooks.com

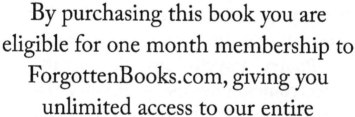

By purchasing this book you are
eligible for one month membership to
ForgottenBooks.com, giving you
unlimited access to our entire
collection of over 1,000,000 titles via
our web site and mobile apps.

To claim your free month visit:

www.forgottenbooks.com/free163675

* Offer is valid for 45 days from date of purchase. Terms and conditions apply.

English
Français
Deutsche
Italiano
Español
Português

www.forgottenbooks.com

Mythology Photography **Fiction**
Fishing Christianity **Art** Cooking
Essays Buddhism Freemasonry
Medicine **Biology** Music **Ancient**
Egypt Evolution Carpentry Physics
Dance Geology **Mathematics** Fitness
Shakespeare **Folklore** Yoga Marketing
Confidence Immortality Biographies
Poetry **Psychology** Witchcraft
Electronics Chemistry History **Law**
Accounting **Philosophy** Anthropology
Alchemy Drama Quantum Mechanics
Atheism Sexual Health **Ancient History**
Entrepreneurship Languages Sport
Paleontology Needlework Islam
Metaphysics Investment Archaeology
Parenting Statistics Criminology
Motivational

TRANSACTIONS

OF THE

AMERICAN PEDIATRIC SOCIETY

TWENTIETH SESSION

HELD AT THE WATER GAP HOUSE, DELAWARE WATER GAP, PENNA.,
ON MAY 25, 26 AND 27, 1908.

———

EDITED BY
LINNÆUS EDFORD LA FÉTRA, M.D.

———

VOLUME XX.

———

REPRINTED FROM
ARCHIVES OF PEDIATRICS
1908–1909

———

E. B. TREAT & CO., PUBLISHERS
241–243 WEST 23D STREET, NEW YORK
1909

A. G. SHERWOOD & CO., PRINTERS,

434 LAFAYETTE STREET,

NEW YORK.

CONTENTS.

PRESIDENTS.

1889. A. JACOBI, M.D.	1899. WM. P. NORTHRUP, M.D.
1890. J. LEWIS SMITH, M.D.	1900. HENRY KOPLIK, M.D.
1891. T. M. ROTCH, M.D.	1901. WM. D. BOOKER, M.D.
1892. WM. OSLER, M.D.	1902. W. S. CHRISTOPHER, M.D.
1893. A. D. BLACKADER, M.D.	1903. J. P. CROZER GRIFFITH, M.D.
1894. JOHN M. KEATING, M.D.	1904. AUGUSTUS CAILLÉ, M.D.
1895. F. FORCHHEIMER, M.D.	1905. C. G. JENNINGS, M.D.
1896. JOSEPH O'DWYER, M.D.	1906. A. JACOBI, M.D.
1897. SAMUEL S. ADAMS, M.D.	1907. B. K. RACHFORD, M.D.
1898. L. EMMETT HOLT, M.D.	1908. C. G. KERLEY, M.D.

1909. CHARLES P. PUTNAM, M.D.

OFFICERS, 1908.

President.......................CHARLES G. KERLEY, M.D.
First Vice-President.............DAVID L. EDSALL, M.D.
Second Vice-President...........HENRY L. K. SHAW, M.D.
Secretary......................SAMUEL S. ADAMS, M.D.
Treasurer......................J. PARK WEST, M.D.
Recorder and Editor.............L. E. LA FÉTRA, M.D.

COUNCIL.

THOMAS MORGAN ROTCH, M.D., Chairman.

F. S. CHURCHILL, M.D.	S. McC. HAMILL, M.D.
L. EMMETT HOLT, M.D.	GEORGE N. ACKER, M.D.
JOHN LOVETT MORSE, M.D.	R. G. FREEMAN, M.D.

MEETING PLACES.

1888. WASHINGTON, D. C. (Organization), September 18.
1889. WASHINGTON and BALTIMORE, September 20 and 21.
1890. NEW YORK, June 3 and 4.
1891. WASHINGTON, September 22 and 25.
1892. BOSTON, May 2, 3 and 4.
1893. WEST POINT, N. Y., May 24, 25 and 26.
1894. WASHINGTON, May 29 and June 1.
1895. VIRGINIA HOT SPRINGS, May 27, 28 and 29.
1896. MONTREAL, May 25, 26 and 27.
1897. WASHINGTON, May 4, 5 and 6.
1898. CINCINNATI, June 1, 2 and 3.
1899. DEER PARK, June 27, 28 and 29.
1900. WASHINGTON, May 1, 2 and 3.
1901. NIAGARA FALLS, May 27, 28 and 29.
1902. BOSTON, May 26, 27 and 28.
1903. WASHINGTON, May 12, 13 and 14.
1904. DETROIT, May 30, 31 and June 1.
1905. LAKE GEORGE, N. Y., June 19, 20 and 21.
1906. ATLANTIC CITY, N. J., May 30, 31 and June 1.
1907. WASHINGTON, May 7, 8 and 9.
1908. DELAWARE WATER GAP, May 25, 26 and 27.
1909. LENOX, MASS., May 27 and 28.

OFFICERS, 1909.

President.......................Charles P. Putnam, M.D.
First Vice-President............Isaac A. Abt, M.D.
Second Vice-President..........Thomas S. Southworth, M.D.
Secretary.......................Samuel S. Adams, M.D.
Treasurer......................J. Park West, M.D.*
Recorder and Editor............L. E. La Fétra, M.D.

COUNCIL.

F. S. Churchill, M.D., Chairman.

L. Emmett Holt, M.D.   George N. Acker, M.D.
John Lovett Morse, M.D.   R. G. Freeman, M.D.
S. McC. Hamill, M.D.   Alfred Hand, Jr., M.D.

MEMBERS.

Abt, Isaac A., M.D...................... .4326, Vincennes Avenue, Chicago
Acker, George N., M.D....................913, Sixteenth Street, Washington
Adams, Samuel S., M.D.......................1, Dupont Circle, Washington
Baines, Allen M., M.D.............................228, Bloor Street, Toronto
Blackader, A. D., M.D ....236, Mountain Street, Montreal
Booker, William D., M.D..............208, West Monument Street, Baltimore
Bovaird, David, Jr., M.D. ....126, West Fifty-eighth St., New York
Buckingham, E. M., M.D.................. ...346, Marlborough Street, Boston
Caillé, Augustus, M.D.....................753, Madison Avenue, New York
Carr, Walter Lester, M.D....... ....68, West Fifty-first Street, New York
Chafin, Henry Dwight, M.D............51, West Fifty-first Street, New York
Churchill, F. S., M.D.......................439, North State Street, Chicago
Cotton, A. C., M.D........................1485, Jackson Boulevard, Chicago
Crandall, Floyd M., M.D............113, West Ninety-fifth Street, New York
Dorning, John, M.D..................124, West Eighty-first Street, New York
Dunn, Charles Hunter, M.D.................220, Marlborough Street, Boston
Eaton, Percival J., M.D............131, N. Highland Avenue, E. E., Pittsburgh
Edsall, David L., M.D................346, South Sixteenth Street, Philadelphia
Fife, Charles A., M.D....................1927, Chestnut Street, Philadelphia
Forchheimer, F., M.D.................Fourth and Sycamore Streets, Cincinnati
Freeman, Rowland G., M.D..... ....205, West Fifty-seventh Street, New York
Graham, E. E., M.D........................1713, Spruce Street, Philadelphia

* Deceased.

GRIFFITH, J. P. CROZER, M.D...............1810, Spruce Street, Philadelphia
HAMILL, S. McC., M.D...............1822, Spruce Street, Philadelphia
HAND, ALFRED, JR., M.D...............1724, Pine Street, Philadelphia
HOLT, L. EMMETT, M.D...............14, West Fifty-fifth Street, New York
HOWLAND, JOHN, M.D...............49, East Fifty-third Street, New York
HUBER, F., M.D...............209, East Seventeenth Street, New York
JACOBI, A., M.D...............19, East Forty-seventh Street, New York
JENNINGS, CHARLES G., M.D...............457, Jefferson Avenue, Detroit
KERLEY, CHARLES G., M.D...............132, West Eighty-first Street, New York
KNOX, J. H. M., M.D...............804, Cathedral Street, Baltimore
KOPLIK, HENRY, M.D...............692, Madison Avenue, New York
LADD, MAYNARD, M.D...............295, Beacon Street, Boston
LA FÉTRA, LINNÆUS E., M.D...............110, East Sixty-second Street, New York
McCOLLOM, JOHN H., M.D...............746, Massachusetts Avenue, Boston
MARTIN, C. F., M.D...............33, Durocher Street, Montreal
MEARA, FRANK S., M.D...............400, West End Avenue, New York
MILLER, D. J. MILTON, M.D...............1700, Pacific Avenue, Atlantic City, N. J.
MORSE, J. LOVETT, M.D...............70, Bay State Road, Boston
NICOLL, MATTHIAS, M.D...............124, East Sixtieth Street, New York
NORTHRUP, WILLIAM P., M.D...............57, East Seventy-ninth Street, New York
PUTNAM, CHARLES P., M.D...............63, Marlborough Street, Boston
RACHFORD, B. K., M.D...............323, Broadway, Cincinnati
ROTCH, THOMAS MORGAN, M.D...............197, Commonwealth Avenue, Boston
RUHRÄH, JOHN, M.D...............839, North Eutaw Street, Baltimore
SAUNDERS, E. W., M.D...............1635, South Grand Avenue, St. Louis, Mo.
SHAW, HENRY L. K., M.D...............198, Washington Avenue, Albany
SNOW, IRVING M., M.D...............476, Franklin Street, Buffalo
SOUTHWORTH, THOMAS S., M.D...............807, Madison Avenue, New York
STARR, LOUIS, M.D...............1818, Rittenhouse Square, Philadelphia
TOWNSEND, CHARLES W., M.D...............76, Marlborough Street, Boston
WENTWORTH, A. H., M.D...............352, Marlborough Street, Boston
WESTCOTT, THOMPSON S., M.D...............1833, Spruce Street, Philadelphia
WILLIAMS, HAROLD, M.D...............528, Beacon Street, Boston
WILSON, W. REYNOLDS, M.D...............1709, Spruce Street, Philadelphia
WINTERS, J. E., M.D...............25, West Thirty-seventh Street, New York

HONORARY MEMBERS.

DR. JOHN THOMPSON...............Edinburgh, Scotland
DR. GEORGE F. STILL...............London, England
DR. HENRY ASHBY...............Manchester, England
DR. O. HEUBNER...............Berlin, Germany
DR. THEODOR ESCHERICH...............Vienna, Austria
DR. WILLIAM OSLER...............Oxford, England
DR. A. BAGINSKY...............Berlin, Germany
DR. V. HUTINEL...............Paris, France
DR. CHARLES RAUCHFUSS...............St. Petersburg, Russia

Deceased.

JOHN A. JEFFRIES, M.D.
Born, September 2, 1859,
Died, March 26, 1892.

THOMAS F. SHERMAN, M.D.
Born, March 17, 1856,
Died, September 26, 1893.

JOHN M. KEATING, M.D.
Born, April 20, 1852,
Died, November 17, 1893.

CHARLES WARRINGTON EARLE, M.D.
Born, 1845,
Died, November 19, 1893.

J. LEWIS SMITH, M.D.
Born, October 15, 1827,
Died, June 9, 1897.

JOSEPH O'DWYER, M.D.
Born, October 12, 1841,
Died, January 7, 1898.

JOHN HENRY FRUITNIGHT, M.D.
Born, November 9, 1851,
Died, December 18, 1900.

FREDERICK A. PACKARD, M.D.
Born, November 17, 1862,
Died, November 1, 1902.

WALTER S. CHRISTOPHER, M.D.
Born, 1859,
Died, March 2, 1905.

LEROY MILTON YALE, M.D.
Born, February 12, 1841.
Died, September 12, 1906.

JAMES PARK WEST, M.D.
Born, June 27, 1858.
Died, June 25, 1908.

MINUTES OF THE TWENTIETH ANNUAL MEETING OF THE AMERICAN PEDIATRIC SOCIETY.

Held at the Water Gap House, Delaware Water Gap, Pa., on May 25 and 26, 1908.

FIRST SESSION, MAY 25TH, 10 A.M.

The meeting was called to order by the President, Dr. C. G. Kerley, who made a brief address of thanks to the Society for the honor of his election as President.

The following members were present: Drs. Isaac A. Abt, Chicago; George N. Acker, Washington; Samuel S. Adams, Washington; Allen Baines, Toronto; E. M. Buckingham, Boston; Augustus Caillé, New York; Walter Lester Carr, New York; Henry Dwight Chapin, New York; F. S. Churchill, Chicago; A. C. Cotton, Chicago; Floyd M. Crandall, New York; John Dorning, New York; Charles Hunter Dunn, Boston; Percival J. Eaton, Pittsburg; David L. Edsall, Philadelphia; Charles A. Fife, Philadelphia; Rowland G. Freeman, New York; E. E. Graham, Philadelphia; J. P. Crozer Griffith, Philadelphia; S. McC. Hamill, Philadelphia; Alfred Hand, Jr., Philadelphia; L. Emmett Holt, New York; John Howland, New York; A. Jacobi, New York; Charles G. Kerley, New York; J. H. Mason Knox, Baltimore; Henry Koplik, New York; L. E. La Fétra, New York; Frank S. Meara, New York; J. Lovett Morse, Boston; William P. Northrup, New York; Charles P. Putnam, Boston; Thomas Morgan Rotch, Boston; John Ruhräh, Baltimore; Irving M. Snow, Buffalo; Thos. S. Southworth, New York; A. H. Wentworth, Boston; J. Park West, Bellaire, O.; W. Reynolds Wilson, Philadelphia; J. E. Winters, New York.

There were present as guests: Drs. Simon Flexner, New York; Frederick H. Bartlett, New York; J. S. Wall and W. W. Wilkinson, of Washington; Frank J. Sladen, Baltimore; Charles A. Gardner, Colorado Springs; O. H. Edwards, Jr., Pittsburg; and Dr. Whiteway, Philadelphia.

Communications of regret at being absent were received from Drs. Booker, of Baltimore, and Jennings, of Detroit.

The minutes of the nineteenth annual meeting were adopted as published in the ARCHIVES OF PEDIATRICS, and Drs. Freeman and Ruhräh were appointed a committee to audit the report of the treasurer.

The President then invited the members and guests of the Society and their wives to enjoy a mountain drive that afternoon.

The following papers were read:

1. Dr. Simon Flexner, New York: "The Serum Treatment of Epidemic Cerebrospinal Meningitis."

2. Dr. Alfred Hand, Jr., Philadelphia: "The Diagnostic Value of the Chemical and Bacteriological Examination of Cerebrospinal Fluid."

3. Drs. J. H. Mason Knox, Jr., and Frank J. Sladen, Baltimore: "Hydrocephalus of Meningococcus Origin, with Remarks on the Serum Treatment."

4. Dr. Charles Hunter Dunn, Boston: "The Serum Treatment of Cerebrospinal Meningitis, with a Report of Cases."

5. Dr. F. S. Churchill, Chicago: "The Serum Treatment of Epidemic Cerebrospinal Meningitis (10 Cases)."

6. Dr. Henry Koplik, New York: "Other Methods of Treatment Compared to the Serum Treatment of Cerebrospinal Meningitis, with a Résumé of Cases of Both Methods of Treatment."

These papers were discussed by Drs. Holt, Rotch, Sladen (guest), Jacobi, Morse, Freeman, Wilkinson (guest), Adams, Kerley; and in closing by Drs. Knox, Dunn, Koplik and Flexner.

MONDAY.—AFTERNOON SESSION.

7. Drs. J. P. Crozer Griffith and R. L. Lavenson, Philadelphia: "Congenital Obliteration of the Esophagus, with the Report of a Case."

8. Dr. Samuel S. Adams, Washington: "Spasmodic Stricture of the Esophagus in an Infant Aged Four Months."

These two papers were discussed by Drs. Caillé, Putnam, Rotch, Jacobi, and, in closing, by Dr. Adams.

9. Dr. Alfred Hand, Jr., Philadelphia: "Exhibition of a Heart with Congenital Defect of the Ventricular Septum, and

Absence of the Pulmonary Artery: Symptoms of Angina Pectoris."

Discussion by Dr. Jacobi.

10. Dr. W. Reynolds Wilson, Philadelphia: "A Simple Method of Circumcision in the Newborn."

Discussed by Dr. A. C. Cotton, Chicago, and, in closing, by the essayist.

11. Dr. J. Park West, Bellaire, O.: "Pyelitis Terminating in Suppurative Nephritis.—Case and Specimen."

Discussion by Drs. Abt, Jacobi and Kerley.

MONDAY.—EVENING SESSION.

12. Dr. Henry Koplik, New York: "Poliomyelitis Anterior Acuta (An Epidemic)."

13. Dr. L. E. La Fétra, New York: "Early Symptoms in the Recent Epidemic of Poliomyelitis."

These papers were discussed by Drs. Holt, Jacobi, Abt, Morse, Kerley, and, in closing, by Dr. Koplik.

14. Dr. E. M. Buckingham, Boston: "Meningitis, Apparently Tubercular, Ending in at Least Temporary Recovery."

15. Dr. John Lovett Morse, Boston: "An Unusual Type of Acute Nephritis in Children."

Discussed by Drs. Koplik, Knox and La Fétra.

TUESDAY, MAY 20TH.—MORNING SESSION.

16. President's address: "Public School Education." By Dr. Charles Gilmore Kerley, New York.

17. Dr. L. Emmett Holt, New York: "Recent Diagnostic Methods in Tuberculosis of Children."

The paper was discussed by Drs. Northrup, Rotch, Caillé, Koplik, Hamill, Wentworth, and, in closing, by the essayist.

18. Dr. William P. Northrup, New York: "Fresh Air in the Treatment of Disease."

19. Dr. E. E. Graham, Philadelphia: "Fresh Air in the Treatment of Disease."

20. Dr. Henry D. Chapin, New York: "A Plan of Dealing with Atrophic Infants."

These three papers were discussed by Drs. Caillé, Jacobi, Freeman, Griffith, Buckingham, Putnam, La Fétra, Kerley, Adams, Churchill, Eaton, Morse, and, in closing, by Drs. Graham, Northrup and Chapin.

TUESDAY.—AFTERNOON SESSION.

21. Dr. Augustus Caillé, New York: "The Need of Postgraduate Instruction in Pediatrics."

22. Thomas Morgan Rotch, Boston: "Modern Laboratory Feeding and the Wide Range of Resources which it Provides."

Discussed by Drs. Holt, Chapin, Caillé, Griffith, Northrup, and, in closing, by Dr. Rotch.

23. Dr. Isaac A. Abt, Chicago: "An Inquiry into the Status of the Kindergarten."

Discussed by Drs. Rotch, Northrup, Churchill, Chapin and Kerley.

24. Drs. Thomas S. Southworth and O. M. Schloss, New York: "The Hard Curds of Infant Stools; Their Origin, Nature and Transformation."

Discussed by Drs. Abt, Morse, Hamill, Northrup, Kerley, and, in closing, by the essayist.

TUESDAY.—EVENING SESSION.

25. Dr. Charles A. Fife, Philadelphia: "Fat and Proteid Content of Top Milks."

Discussed by Drs. Griffith, Chapin, Southworth, Eaton, and, in closing, by the essayist.

26. Drs. J. H. Mason Knox and J. C. Meakins, Baltimore: "The Urinary Findings in a Series of Infants Suffering from Intestinal Infection."

Discussed by Dr. Abt.

The following papers were read by title:—

"Congenital Hypertrophic Stenosis of the Pylorus—Case," by John Dorning, M.D., New York.

"Recurring Empyema"; "Abscess of Lung due to Wire Nail Two Inches Long in Right Bronchus; Operation; Recovery, with Surgical Comments by Dr. H. M. Silver," by Francis Huber, M.D., New York.

"An Investigation of the Effects of Various Milk Modifiers

upon the Gastric Digestion of Infants," by L. Emmett Holt, M.D., and Thomas W. Clarke, M.D., New York.

"Some Observations Regarding a Fourth Exanthem—the So-called Duke's Disease," by A. C. Cotton, M.D., Chicago.

EXECUTIVE SESSION.—10 P.M.

The special Committee on Revision of the Constitution made its report, which was accepted and, with certain amendments, adopted.

The report of the Council was read by Dr. Rotch, and its recommendations adopted, as follows:

As officers for the ensuing year there were elected:

President, Dr. Charles P. Putnam, Boston.

First Vice-President, Dr. Isaac A. Abt, Chicago.

Second Vice-President, Dr. Thos. S. Southworth, New York.

Secretary, Dr. Samuel S. Adams, Washington.

Treasurer, Dr. J. Park West, Bellaire, O.

Recorder, Dr. L. E. La Fétra, New York.

As member of the Council to take the place of Dr. Rotch, retiring, Dr. Alfred Hand, Jr. As member of the Executive Committee, Congress of American Physicians and Surgeons, Dr. A. Jacobi; alternate, Dr. J. P. Crozer Griffith.

Elected to membership: Dr. Matthias Nicoll, Jr., New York.

Elected to honorary membership: Dr. Charles Rauchfuss, St. Petersburg, Russia.

The Secretary reported that Prof. Schlossman, of Düsseldorf, had been invited to be present at the meeting, but had sent a letter declining and expressing his appreciation of the honor.

The report of the Treasurer was reported correct by the Auditing Committee, Drs. Freeman and Ruhräh.

The annual assessment for dues was made $10.

It was decided to hold the next annual meeting at Lenox, Mass., on May 27 and 28, 1909.

The Secretary moved a vote of thanks to the President for one of the most successful meetings the Society had ever had, and this was accordingly given.

SAMUEL S. ADAMS, M.D.,
Secretary.
LINNÆUS EDFORD LA FÉTRA, M.D.,
Recorder.

PUBLIC SCHOOL EDUCATION.

BY CHARLES GILMORE KERLEY, M.D.,
New York.

The education of a child, taken in a broad sense, "comprehends all that disciplines and enlightens the understanding, cultivates the taste and forms the manners and habits."* It means a preparation, a means to the end of fitting the child for a field of activity whereby his own life may be made more satisfactory to himself and of the most use to the State.

In order to bring this about, the curriculum must include instruction other than that which relates to things purely academic. The child must be taught how to live. This constitutes knowledge just as fully as an acquaintance with arithmetic or geography constitutes knowledge, and its acquirement calls for an exercise of those higher mental processes which develop the reasoning faculties. If we have the best interests of the child at heart we must, as Bacon puts it, "determine the relative value of knowledges." "How to live. That is the essential question. Not how to live in the mere material sense, but in the wider sense; the general problem which comprehends every special problem, is the right ruling of conduct in all directions and under all circumstances. In what way to treat the body; in what way to treat the mind; in what way to behave as a citizen; in what way to utilize all those sources of happiness which nature supplies. How to use all our faculties to the greatest advantage to ourselves and to others. How to live completely. To prepare us for complete living is the function which education has to discharge, and the only rational mode of judging of any educational course is the judging in what degree it discharges such functions."†

Our subject will be considered from two standpoints—that which relates to the child's physical, and that which relates to his mental, development.

In the United States today there are 18,000,000 children in attendance at the public schools. The school year has been increased from three months to ten months. Owing to changed con-

---

* Standard Dictionary.
† Herbert Spencer.

ditions of living in all classes, as a result of stress and competition, of social duties and amusements, or to indifference and indolence, parents see comparatively little of their children—much less than fifty, twenty-five or twenty years ago. The chief control of the child has been transferred from the home to the school, which means that the duties and responsibilities of the public school have increased tremendously.

An immense majority of these 18,000,000 children will complete their schooling between the fourteenth and the sixteenth year. They will pass out of the school door to take up the world's work. What do they know? How are they prepared for complete living? I have known a great many boys and girls who completed the grammar and high school courses. I have followed them through the years of their study and have watched their later lives. The child under fourteen years of age is by law, in New York State, required to go to school. If not, he is a truant, and his parents are subjected to a fine or other discipline. The State takes the child from his game, from the street, from the park, or from the field, puts him into the school and demands that he remain there five hours a day, five days in a week.

What is the child's treatment in the school? First, as relates to his physical well-being? In the last annual report of the Superintendent of Schools of New York City, the superintendent, Dr. Maxwell, referring to the manner in which the city cares for both the well and defective school children, writes as follows:—

"Sitting several hours a day at a desk which may not be hygienically constructed increases such diseases as curvature of the spine and often produces faults of posture, which the physical exercises of the class-room and the gymnasium barely avail to counteract. Defects in eyesight are certainly aggravated, as will presently be shown, by the work of the class-room. In short, though the school is doing what it may, with its present resources, to neutralize the evil effects of urban life upon children, yet these resources are inadequate, because they do little or nothing for those children who are suffering from a physical defect."

Six hundred thousand children in New York City schools are being compelled to read more or less for five hours a day in artificially lighted buildings without any consultation or investigation being made from the medical standpoint as to the effects.*

---

* Dr. Luther H. Gulick.

In the New York City schools, after the tenth year, there is practically no recreation period between nine and twelve or between one and three o'clock. Nominally there is a twenty-minute period, but this is usually taken up with other duties. Physical training comprises a part of the curriculum, but comparatively few children can avail themselves of it, because of lack of time or of physical defects which would render such exercises of no value.

"It appears, from the reports of the Board of Health, that over 30 per cent. of the children in our schools have a degree of eye-deformity sufficiently severe to interfere with their progress from grade to grade. It is reported, from sources that are apparently trustworthy, that in some schools a very much larger percentage than this of children who have been in school for two years or more have such eye-deformities and that this is due to the deficient light in these buildings. These eye-deformities increase from year to year throughout school life with such regularity that it is almost possible to place a certain grade by reporting upon the percentage of eye-deformity found among its members."*

As a general proposition there should be no choice between health and education; only that education is effective which is founded upon, and which secures, good health.

The superintendent's suggestion, that a department of hygiene be organized to coöperate with the Board of Education, is most timely. Such a board should be made up of a skilled oculist, an orthopedist, a laryngologist, a pediatrist and a sanitarian, who should be given power to arrange suitable type and printing for the different ages, to consider problems of ventilation and lighting, of posture, of vision. of the nose and throat, of nutrition and growth and of general hygiene and to direct the recreation periods. A standard of control—a health clearing-house—should be established as to what would be considered the normal requirements for the various ages.

Obviously oculists, and other specially trained physicians only, are competent to direct the various means of maintaining and restoring health to the school child, and as such should constitute an Advisory Board to the Board of Education and the City. The contagious disease should remain where it is, in control of

---

* Dr. Gulick, Ninth Annual Report, Superintendent of Schools. New York City.

the Health Department, but general medical inspection should be under the control of this Board of Hygiene.

"At a recent physical examination in Minneapolis, Minn., it is reported that only 17 per cent. of the children were defective. Boston reports 54 per cent., New York 60 per cent. and Sioux City 80 per cent. The range in eyesight is about the same. Columbus, O., reports about 25 per cent., New York about 30 per cent., while Wellesley, Mass., reports 63 per cent."*

Obviously such statistics are without value, excepting to prove that a large percentage of children are defective, and to suggest the necessity of establishing a standard that will apply to all schools.

A review of the work of medical inspection and of sanitary regulations in general is of interest.*   The first regular medical inspector in America was Dr. Morreau Morris, who was appointed in New York in 1892.   There is but one state (Massachusetts) which has a law providing for medical inspection in all the schools.   Only sixteen states provide for fire-escapes and fire protection.   Only Massachusetts and Connecticut have established a standard of ventilation and require its enforcement. Kentucky alone provides standards for lighting, floor spaces, air spaces, seating and water supply.   Only one-third of the states compel vaccination.   In the great State of Indiana there is no medical inspection.   The Secretary of the State Board of Health of Iowa has recently published an article against medical inspection.

The general neglect and haphazard methods of handling this vitally important matter; the conflicting views and opinions as evidenced by the laws in operation, and by the absence of laws, demand that the subject of school hygiene, and of education of the young in general, be placed under Federal, instead of State, control, even if a constitutional amendment is required to bring it about.   If the figures given as related to defectives are true, the United States is sustaining much financial loss and is greatly handicapped in attempting to educate children who are in such a physical condition that they will not profit by the instruction offered.   The expense to the State of maintaining a child in school one day is twenty-four cents.   The necessity of helping this situation, of stopping this waste, emphasizes the necessity of

---

* Dr. Gulick.

wise medical guidance. The Americanizing of the large alien population involves their receiving new habits of life with reference to health and the care of their own children, and demands the exercise of much care and labor by physicians.

A large fraction of the children that are in our city schools either themselves come from non-English-speaking countries or are children of those who come from these countries. That a large proportion of the population of our great cities is made up of persons from foreign parentage is not generally realized. The facts as told in the late census in regard to some of our leading cities are as follows:—

POPULATION OF NATIVE AND FOREIGN PARENTAGE IN 1900.

City.	Per Cent. Foreign.
Boston	77.2
Chicago	77.4
Detroit	77.4
Jersey City	70.5
Milwaukee	82.7
Newark	82.8
New York	76.9
St. Paul	72.6
San Francisco	82.1

After giving the child reasonable sanitary accommodations, and after using means to place him, and keep him, in the best physical condition, we would beg leave to suggest certain changes in the curriculum. We would have the boy and girl who are to go out in life at the fourteenth or fifteenth year of age taught reading and penmanship, geography, history and arithmetic, and given industrial and trade instruction. These are essentials as necessary to complete living and will be useful throughout the life of the individual. The curriculum of the elementary and high schools, however, includes more than these. It includes modern languages, music, Greek and Spanish history, zoology, commercial law, etc. We have no criticism to offer against these studies, excepting that they are non-essentials and crowd out other instruction which comprehends the essential. And, further, such studies are time wasted for the great majority, who will quit school life at the fourteenth or fifteenth year.

Among the essentials I would include religion. Any preparation for life is incomplete without a reasonable conception of its ethical principles. Many children never attend Sunday-school. In many instances, religious instruction is not given in the home, although, as a necessity to complete living, it comprises an important part of education and should be taught in the school. I realize that this is a most delicate and difficult matter to deal with, but it must be solved. There is no question but that the need exists. Departmental work is carried on in all schools. The State forces attendance at the schools and dictates to a considerable degree the course of study. It should provide religious instruction for those who want it, at least in all large cities where it is needed most. Protestants (and I am one) need it the most, because the home training is weaker than in the other faiths; at least, this is my observation.

The necessity for a sound religious training for the development of rational religious conviction is demonstrated in the spread of the Christian Science dogma, the creation of a mind diseased, to which thousands are adherents. These converts are rarely of the Catholic or the Hebrew faith.

Social Prophylaxis.—Morrow, in the *Maryland Medical Journal,* of September, 1907, states that competent European observers agree that 75 per cent. of the adult population have, or have had, gonorrhea, and that from 10 to 18 per cent. contract syphilis. He believes it conservative to state that the morbidity from both these infections in this country would be present in 60 per cent. of the male population. Gynecologists tell us that from 60 to 80 per cent. (different writers varying somewhat) of the acute inflammatory pelvic disorders in women are due to gonorrhea innocently acquired, and that 35 per cent. of all operative pelvic conditions in women have the gonococcus as the etiological factor. Thirty per cent. of the cases of blindness are attributed to the gonococcus, the infection being acquired at birth. It is estimated that 50 per cent. of the cases of gonorrhea in men are contracted before the twentieth year, and in practically all instances the patient possesses little or no knowledge as to the gravity to himself or the far-reaching and terrible consequences to others.

An important feature in the boy's education is here neglected.

"The ideal of a good education to which most parents cling is one which entirely ignores the existence of sex, the most important feature of life. Through a lack of courage, or through a sense of false modesty, the system of generation is looked upon as a system of shame. This impression is so fixed and grounded in the mind of youth that it is apt to dominate his mental attitude throughout life. This sex instruction, to their sons so inauspiciously begun, is then committed to haphazard sources, to servants, to old or dissolute companions, and quack literature."*

It is the duty of the medical profession, who are in a position to appreciate the necessity of such instruction, to insist that it be carried on through the proper channels, the schools, by ways and means which seem best for those expert in training the young.

Let it be taught what constitutes morality, but do not neglect the physical side of the subject. The possible consequences of transgression should also be known. I have known three girls who became pregnant in the thirteenth year and not one of them knew the nature of the sex relation.

It is not claimed that proper instruction along the above lines would remedy all the evils referred to, but for right living a knowledge as to what constitutes it is required, and when the impress is made in the right way upon the impressionable mind of youth, much good will result, and we would not hear it said, as I have heard it time and again, "I did not know that such things were."

Alcohol and Narcotics.—One of the great scourges of the earth is intemperance in the use of alcohol. This is a practice which is the direct or indirect cause of more crime, poverty, diseases and untimely death than any other one factor, and yet it is passed over in our public institutions of learning with but meagre attention, in spite of the fact that laws exist in all the states which require that such instruction shall be given. It is interesting to note that these laws, making such study compulsory, have been secured almost wholly by the efforts of women, led by the late Mrs. Mary H. Hunt, of Boston, who for twenty years gave her whole time and fortune to the task. Physicians as a body have done but little in this direction.

I judge that this study is neglected from the knowledge of the subject possessed by the New York City finished product at the fifteenth or sixteenth year of age. In order to give the child what he has a right to demand, and for his own interest

---

* Morrow.

and his own protection, he should know the effects of alcohol, immediate and remote, as well as he knows the multiplication table. I am not advocating prohibition, or that it be taught. I speak for the boy and girl in a personal and selfish sense only.

An intimate association with a great many people in an active life for many years has resulted in the formation of a few additional convictions regarding educational matters. One conviction is that we are being educated to a danger point. State colleges and schools, semi-private and so-called private, are founded and endowed. Scholarships are supplied, not because of the law of supply and demand, but because some rich man or woman desires to ease a conscience or erect a lasting monument, with the result of making a certain proportion of the incompetent still more unfit. The next step which is in order, and not far in the distance, will be the offering of gratuities to students because students must be had. This factor in the life of the body politic, together with a spirit that exists in our public schools and in schools generally, is doing much to disorganize society. This spirit or sentiment is a species of madness and is a distinct Americanism. It is the desire for end results. It is the American spirit of "getting there" regardless of the method. We see it in our public life. We have all had ample demonstration of its operative possibilities in the business and financial world during the past year. This sentiment in the schools has been deplored by as eminent a teacher as Dr. J. E. Russell, of the New York Teachers College. This system of instruction appears to consist of a process of imparting specific information which is to be remembered, the end results being answers to questions. Actual knowledge, founded and acquired through processes of the reasoning faculties, is not particularly apparent in the finished product. I know not a few who show a lack of mental force, defective concentration and an absence of knowledge which should have been acquired during the training of this higher function.

The system of prizes and rewards for the best recitations, or set of answers in a given subject, is a bad one, as it overtaxes the pupil and it usually means a matter of memory. For certain excellence at recitation a boy patient, whom I was obliged to take out of a private school, received daily a red card. When he had five red cards he received a large yellow card. I asked him what the yellow card stood for. He did not know. He had worked so hard to get these yellow cards, the significance of which he did not know, that I was obliged to take him from school. He could scarcely hold a pack of these yellow cards in his hands because of the chorea which was present.

By suggestion and encouragement, if not by direct advice, the young of our schools are under the stress of a constant incentive to strain after greatness. Emulation is in the school air. Every boy in some way is made to believe that in him is the metal from which Presidents of the United States are fashioned; that out of such material as the great financiers, lawyers, physicians and teachers are moulded; that he ought to be great, and if he gets his lessons by some means or other, he is taking his first step toward so-called greatness. I look upon it as most unfortunate for the boys of this country that Abraham Lincoln split rails and was born in a log-cabin; that General Grant was a tanner; that Garfield drove mules before a canal boat, and that Russell Sage sold newspapers. In defence of this teaching it is claimed that high ideals should be placed before the young. The highest ideals do not have end results in the acquirement of wealth or power or position. Bringing a child up in an atmosphere thus charged is the inevitable cause of much disappointment, suicide and life failures, and for the reason that it is impossible to build a $10,000, $20,000 or $40,000 a year intellect in a two-dollar a day brain. This spirit, with the encouragement from all sources —endowments, scholarships and rich men's colleges—toward so-called higher education, induces youths to spend years in striving and end in failure more or less complete. This over-education of the unfit brings forth tastes, habits and desires of which he should not know, and is the cause of more thieving, gambling and all around dishonesty than is well appreciated. When position and wealth or reasonable competency do not follow by legitimate means, others are readily seized upon.

The labor question in this country is a most serious one. In times of usual prosperity it is well-nigh impossible to get workmen. During building operations which I had under way a few years ago, from $5 to $8 a day for a so-called eight-hour day was paid. In periods of depression, skilled laborers fare no worse than others. Among the boys whom I have known intimately during the past twenty years, sons of carpenters, shoemakers, plumbers, bricklayers, etc., I have known not one who wished his occupation to be that of his father. These boys would all be lawyers, bank presidents, physicians, etc., and, sorry to relate, some of them became lawyers or physicians. No bank presidents, but poorly paid bookkeepers they are today. None would be a wage-earner with the father, because of the efforts to make him think above it. All the professions are overcrowded with the disappointed unfit. I know physicians whose income from their practice is less than $1,000 a year. Ten per cent. of those graduated in medicine fail to make a living and seek other occupation. A few years ago, when I was experiencing difficulty in getting workmen at $5 a day, a lawyer friend advertised in a daily paper for clerks somewhat familiar with legal work, to do copying of a certain nature at a salary of $8 a week. Among those who applied were seventeen lawyers, who had been admitted to the bar of New York State. The great majority of bookkeepers, clerks and small business men and many male teachers have less earning capacity than the man with a trade.

I would impress upon teachers and the Board of Education this thought: "That labor is the inevitable lot of the majority, and that the best education is that which makes labor the most productive." For the boy who is to go out and become a member of the working class, as millions must, I would have inserted somewhere in the curriculum, somewhere between the Spanish history period and the elocution period, a few minutes devoted to a talk on honest toil and the nobility of labor, and that the only dishonorable work is that which is badly done. I would have boys taught reading, writing and arithmetic and the rudiments of a trade. Somewhere between the zoology and commercial law period I would have the girl who is to bring up a family of children, and who will have to do her own housework, get more than a passing glance at physiology, cooking, sewing and food values.

At this moment these 18,000,000 boys and girls in the public schools are not being furnished the physical advantages and protection that they have a right to demand. They are not being taught how to live.

And if we judge of our public school educational course according to the degree with which it discharges its function, we are forced to admit that it fails in its function.

AN ANALYSIS OF FOUR HUNDRED CASES OF EPIDEMIC MENINGITIS TREATED WITH THE ANTIMENINGITIS SERUM.

BY SIMON FLEXNER, M.D.,

AND

JAMES W. JOBLING, M.D.,

New York.

(From the Rockefeller Institute for Medical Research, New York.)

We have already reported concerning the effects of the employment of an antimeningitis serum, prepared in the horse by inoculation of *diplococcus intracellularis* and its products, upon the course and termination of a small number of cases of epidemic meningitis.* The results first presented were, on the whole, so satisfactory that we believed the employment of the serum on wider scale not only justified but clearly called for; and we are now in position to present a second series of figures which are based upon an analysis of about 400 cases of epidemic meningitis in which the serum has been used.

The cases of meningitis upon which this analysis rests have arisen in different and widely separated parts of the United States and Canada, and in Great Britain. They have occurred sometimes as small epidemics, as in Castalia and Akron, O., in Porterville, Cal., and, possibly, in other places in the United States, and in Belfast, Ireland, and Edinburgh, Scotland; and sometimes as sporadic outbreaks of considerable extent, as in Cleveland, Boston, Baltimore, Cincinnati and Philadelphia. Moreover, it is now evident that so-called epidemic meningitis is widely prevalent throughout the United States, and it would appear to be questionable whether any parts are really free from the disease. In view of the fact that we have demanded that the bacteriological diagnosis be made in every case of meningitis for which we have supplied the serum, and which we have accepted for our analysis, and that in doubtful instances we have

---

* Journal of Experimental Medicine, 1908, x, No. 1. Independent publications have been made by Robb, British Medical Journal, February 15, 1908; by Dunn, Boston Medical and Surgical Journal, March 19, 1908; and by Chase and Hunt, Archives of Clinical Medicine, April, 1908.

ourselves examined slides and sometimes cultures prepared from the spinal exudates, we can speak with positiveness upon this important subject.

It is an important matter, and one to be carefully pondered, whether the wide distribution of sporadic epidemic meningitis in the United States is the outcome and residue of the epidemic that raged in New York and vicinity from 1905 to 1907, or whether the disease tends to exist and has long existed in a sporadic state in this country, from which the severe epidemic outbreaks have occasionally taken their origin. There is some reason to suppose that the diagnosis of sporadically occurring cases of the disease may fail to be made unless attention is specially directed to the unusual symptoms by the simultaneous occurrence of several such cases, or by a wider publicity which the disease sometimes attains as through the existence of obvious epidemic foci, or, as in the present instance, by the interest excited by the publications relating to the antimeningitis serum.

The analysis which is to be presented is based upon histories of cases of epidemic meningitis in which the diagnosis has been established by bacteriological examinations as well as by the usual clinical tests. The histories have been supplied by physicians in hospitals and in private practice, who have employed the serum. It will not be possible in this place to acknowledge duly and by name the physicians who so generously gave their time to the study of the effects of the serum. But we hope soon to publish a full report of this investigation, when the awarding of due credit will be attempted.*

In making up the figures upon which the tabulations are based, account has been taken of the ages of the patients, the period of the disease at which the serum was first injected, the number of injections of the serum made, the dosage of the serum, the effects on the temperature, and the subjective and objective symptoms of the disease, upon the number and viability of the diplococcus in the spinal exudate, the general leukocytosis, the duration of the fever and other symptoms, the manner of recovery —that is, whether by slow improvement or lysis, or by abrupt termination of the symptoms or crisis—and some other details of the disease. Not all the points that have been developed can be brought out in this shorter article. But we wish to state that

---

* To appear in Journal of Experimental Medicine, 1908, x, No. 5.

in one way only has any selection of cases been made, namely, that all cases which survived the first dose of serum less than twenty-four hours have been excluded from the tabulations. We consider that it may be accepted as probable that any marked benefit which the serum may be assumed to exert could hardly be effectively exhibited before the first twenty-four-hour period following its administration had elapsed. It has chanced that of the histories here analyzed the eliminations include chiefly cases which were moribund at the time of their admission to hospitals and the first serum injections and in which the survival was often only a few hours—one hour to five or six hours—and, in addition, a certain although small number of rapidly fatal fulminating cases.

Result According to the Ages of the Patients.—The total number of cases subjected to tabulation is 393.* The total number of recoveries among these cases was 295 and the total number of deaths 98. Hence, there was 75 per cent. of recoveries and 25 per cent. of deaths. Tabulated according to the ages of the patients, the following is the result obtained:—

	No. of Cases.	Recovered.	Died.	Died.
Under 1 year	22	11	11	50 per cent.
Between 1 and 2 years	19	11	8	42.1 " "
" 2 " 5 "	68	52	16	23.5 " "
" 5 " 10 "	79	70	9	11.4 " "
" 10 " 20 "	105	80	25	23.8 " "
Over 20 years	87	64	23	26.4 " "
Age not given	13	7	6	46.1 " "

The youngest child who recovered was one month old. The latest case of the disease, in a child under one year of age, which was treated, was in its fourth month when the injections were begun: the child died. The highest mortality was among cases over twenty years of age, which can, we think, be explained in part by the fact that a larger number were treated by scattered physicians who had no experience with the serum. If this is not the reason, and adults past twenty are less subject to the action of the serum than younger persons, the fact will, of course, come out finally; but with one exception (Cincinnati), wherever a

---

* Representing the number after the moribund and fulminating cases have been subtracted.

series of cases of these ages had been treated by one observer, the percentage of recoveries to deaths has been high. (Johns Hopkins Hospital, Baltimore, Cleveland, Belfast, Ireland.)

Results According to the Period of Injection.—We have also analyzed the histories according to the earliest period of the disease at which the injection of the serum was begun. Not all the histories are perfectly definite on this point, and hence we have used in the analysis only those that are definite. In not a few cases the onset of the disease was insidious and the prodromata appear to have been indefinite and more or less overlooked. At other times, and this seems to have been the more frequent experience, the onset was abrupt, so that no special doubt surrounded the beginning of the disease. Under the circumstances, therefore, the danger is that the period elapsing between the onset and the symptoms of the disease, their recognition, the first serum injection, will be calculated too short rather than too long. It is very rare, except in the fulminant cases, that one can assure himself that he is dealing with the disease on the first day of its existence.

The histories of 361 cases were sufficiently explicit to enable us to approximate the periods in which the first serum injection was made. We have arbitrarily chosen the three periods that follow in which to group the cases:—

Period of Injection of Serum.	No. of Cases.	Recovered.	Died.	Died.
First to third day	123	107	16	16.5 per cent.
Fourth to seventh day.	126	96	30	23.8 " "
Later than seventh day	112	73	39	35 " "

In spite of the uncertainties surrounding the period of onset of the symptoms which affect the accuracy of the calculation of the period, the beneficial influence of early injection is rendered sufficiently obvious by the table. The period embraced in the last group is, of course, highly irregular, since not a few cases came under treatment when they were in a semi-chronic, or chronic, state after many weeks of illness. On the whole, therefore, the outlook even for the latter class of cases is not wholly discouraging; and, indeed, we are of the opinion that so long as the diplococcus is still present in the meningeal exudate and the mechanical damage to the anatomical structure is not irreparable, the employment of the serum holds out hope of considerable benefit.

Manner of Termination of the Symptoms.—The histories have been sufficiently explicit in 273 instances to enable us to determine the manner in which the disease terminated, that is, whether by lysis or crisis. We do not think that our decisions on this point have been uniformly correct and the figures are given, therefore, merely as an approximation of what may be found later to be the true figures. Of the 270 cases described in the histories, 200 terminated by lysis and 73 by crisis. Hence we have assumed that from 25 per cent. to 30 per cent. of the cases treated with the serum terminated abruptly in the manner to which we previously applied the term "crisis."

Closely connected with the question of the manner of termination of the symptoms is the question of the duration of the active symptoms of the disease in serum-treated as compared with non-serum-treated cases. Without entering into a discussion of this point we wish to state that we have analyzed 228 histories of recovered patients with reference to the duration of the active symptoms and found the period to be about eleven days.

Influence on Diplococci, Spinal Exudate and Leukocytosis.— In our first publication on the serum treatment of epidemic meningitis we drew attention to a fact, which impressed us as remarkable and significant, namely, that very soon after the serum injections were begun the diplococci tended to be greatly reduced in numbers, to disappear from the fluid part of the exudate, to become wholly intracellular (unless they were now entirely absent), to present certain changes in appearance, as swelling and fragmentation, and to stain diffusely and indistinctly, and co-incidentally to lose viability in cultures. The later and far wider experience has tended to confirm the views we first expressed based on the effects observed; and while exceptions occur in which the diplococci disappear or become engulfed and change in morphology or lose viability more slowly, yet the general fact seems securely established. There seems little doubt that part of the beneficial effect of the serum injections must arise from the restriction of multiplication and from the greater phagocytosis of the diplococci.

Attention was previously directed to the rapidity with which the exudate in the meninges loses turbidity under the influence of the serum injections. This fact has been noted again and again in the subsequent cases treated with the serum. Indeed, it would now appear as if the fear we expressed, that the cases with strictly purulent exudates might be less amenable to the action of the serum, was premature. A fair number of cases in which the notes state the spinal exudate to have been purulent have recovered, and the rapid clearing of the exudate was observed even in them. Whether there is complete anatomical restitution of the meninges in these cases can only be determined by postmortem examinations, but that complete functional restoration can take place may be regarded as certain.

Closely connected with the rapidity with which the cerebrospinal exudate loses pus cells and returns to a limpid condition, is the state of the general leukocytes of the blood. If the inflammatory emigration into the meninges is arrested, then the number of circulating leukocytes should tend rapidly to return to the normal. The facts at hand, based upon many counts of the circulating leukocytes before the injections of serum were begun, and afterward at regular intervals, show, as was to be expected, a fall, often very rapid and even critical, in the number of leukocytes in the general blood stream with which the disappearance of the diplococci and the clearing of the spinal exudate are correlated.

The reverse of the phenomena here mentioned is encountered in those cases not responding to the serum, or responding imperfectly, in which death is the result. Although the data bearing on this topic at our command are less numerous and perfect than the other, yet the general statement can be made that the diplococci, the spinal exudate, and the circulating leukocytes are less influenced in the resistant cases, and that progressive increase in turbidity of the exudate and rise in leukocytosis, and greater persistence of the diplococci with retention of viability after several injections of the serum, are unfavorable indications.

The data at hand, bearing on the meningeal phenomena that precede and attend the relapses so far as diplococci, exudate and leukocytosis go, are also imperfect. Here, again, the general statement can be made that the relapses are attended or ushered in by increased exudation of leukocytes into the meninges, higher systemic leukocytosis, and reappearance of, or increase in, the numbers of diplococci, although the diplococci may not regain power to grow outside the body in cultures. Relapses, in the course of the treatment, are not very frequent and rarely has the case terminated fatally during relapse when the treatment with the serum has been resumed without delay and vigorously pushed.

There remains one more topic to be mentioned. The indications given by the first·series of serum-treated cases were to the effect that in the great majority of instances recovery from the disease would be complete. The facts brought out by the far larger series of cases on which this article is based, confirm the earlier view which we expressed. The number of complications which arose in them was small, and the only persistent defect noted was deafness. This lamentable condition occurred in a few instances only, and it was, more often than not, noted early in the disease before the serum injections were begun.

PAPER ON THE SERUM TREATMENT OF MENIN-GOCOCCIC MENINGITIS.

BY FRANK S. CHURCHILL, M.D.

I have had the opportunity to watch the effect of the Flexner antimeningitic serum upon 11 cases of undoubted meningitis—9 of the meningococcic type, 2 undetermined. Four of these have died—the 2 undetermined cases and 2 of the meningococcic type. Thus, 7 of the 9 cases of the latter variety have recovered, all without serious sequelæ.

All the cases were clinically meningitis and a diagnosis of the gross lesion could have been made without lumbar puncture, though, of course, not the type of the disease present. The chief interest in the cases has, of course, been in noting the effect of the serum. This has been striking. It has been noted upon the general condition of the patient, upon the temperature and leukocyte curves, upon the color and contents of the spinal fluid.

Usually the first effect noticed clinically has been the change in the patient's mentality. He would seem brighter and more rational after the first, second or third dose of the serum, as the case might be, and this improvement continued steadily until the patient was well. It was a curious sight to see the patient lying in bed with head markedly retracted, yet perfectly quiet and without pain, interested in his surroundings, for the rigidities persisted after the mental state began to clear up. Kernig's sign was particularly persistent in some cases.

The leukocyte curve was an interesting phenomenon. There was, of course, a considerable leukocytosis at the outset of treatment, but after the use of the serum there was almost invariably a drop in the leukocyte curve, together with a drop in the temperature curve.

The effect of the serum upon the spinal fluid was striking. At the outset of the disease the fluid was, of course, cloudy; in 2 cases, purulent. Examination of the first specimen of fluid obtained generally showed considerable numbers of leukocytes of the polymorphonuclear variety and also meningococci, varying in numbers with the intensity of the disease. Subsequent punctures showed a fluid less cloudy, and, by actual count, a diminishing number of cells and organisms. The latter were found both extra- and intracellular.

In view of what we now know of this antimeningitic serum, I believe we are justified in this opinion: given a case, evidently meningitis, it is our duty to do a lumbar puncture, and if we obtain a cloudy fluid to inject the serum at once into the spinal canal, subsequent injections being determined by the results of the bacteriological examination of the spinal fluid. If this show the presence of the meningococcus, the serum should be repeated every day for three or four days if necessary. If relapses occur, we should resort to the serum again.

THE SERUM TREATMENT OF EPIDEMIC CEREBRO-SPINAL MENINGITIS, BASED ON A SERIES OF FORTY CONSECUTIVE CASES.

BY CHARLES HUNTER DUNN, M.D.,

Boston, Mass.

The report is based on a series of 40 consecutive cases of epidemic cerebrospinal meningitis, treated with Dr. Flexner's antimeningitis serum. All cases in which the diplococcus intracellularis' was found in the cerebrospinal fluid, without regard to the type of case or the stage of the disease, are included in the series. The antiserum was administered in all cases by injection into the cerebrospinal canal according to the technic recommended by Dr. Flexner and described in a previous publication. As soon as a suspected case was reported to me, lumbar puncture was at once performed. If the cerebrospinal fluid obtained was cloudy, the antiserum was injected at once, without waiting for the bacteriologic examination of the cerebrospinal fluid, and if fluid was clear no antiserum was given until subsequent examination revealed the presence of the diplococcus intracellularis.

In those cases in which a rapid and marked improvement in the symptoms occurred after the first injection, accompanied by a permanent fall of temperature to the normal, no further injection was given. In those cases in which this did not occur, the injections were repeated daily until nervous and subjective symptoms were completely relieved and the temperature had reached the normal, or until four doses had been given. In resistant or relapsing cases further doses were given according to circumstances. The routine dose was 30 c.c.; in many instances larger doses were given, the maximum being 45 c.c. In some instances, when the amount of fluid obtained was small, and in all instances when too great an increase of intradural pressure was feared, smaller amounts were injected, the minimum being 10 c.c. This was the general routine; there were some exceptions.

The serum has been used in 45 cases of epidemic cerebrospinal meningitis, but cases still pending are not included in the series. Of the 40 finished cases nine patients have died and thirty-one have recovered. This is a mortality of 22.5 per cent. and a rate of recovery of 77.5 per cent. Of the 31 cases in which the patients recovered, two were left with sequelæ, one being deaf and one both blind and deaf. The recovery was complete in 29 cases, or in 72.5 per cent.

The type of disease prevailing this year in Boston and vicinity was no milder than that which prevails every year.

I have not been able, for purposes of comparison, to collect enough cases treated in Boston and vicinity this year without the antiserum. It is possible, however, to compare the mortality at the Children's Hospital this year under the use of the antiserum with the mortality in other years under other methods of treatment, as sufficient cases have been treated in this hospital each year to afford a basis for such a comparison. While the number of cases treated each year varies, the average yearly number for the last ten years is twenty. This comparison also throws light on the comparative value of the treatment with the antiserum and of other methods.

It appears that the lowest mortality of any year before this was 58 per cent., and that it varied between 58 per cent. and 80 per cent., but that this year, under the use of the Flexner antiserum, the mortality has shown a remarkable drop to only 19 per cent.

The 9 fatal cases in the series throw a certain amount of light on the limitations of the value of the serum. Of these nine, five were cases seen late in the course of the disease, at a time when the patients were in the well-known chronic stage, unconscious, and without fever or active symptoms. In one of these the serum was not given until the patient was actually moribund. Of the other 4 cases, one was of the fulminating type, one a very severe case, and one patient died of an intercurrent bronchopneumonia, coming on after the temperature had come down to normal and all meningeal symptoms had subsided. The last case was one of average severity, in which the serum appeared to produce a slight improvement in the beginning, but which later appeared uninfluenced by the antiserum, advanced into the chronic stage, and a fatal result ensued after many weeks of illness.

My belief in the great value of the Flexner antimeningitis serum is based not chiefly on its apparent effect on the mortality of the disease, but on the very marked and striking effect which

its use appears to produce in individual cases. It so modifies and
changes the course of the disease as to present a very sharp contrast with the course usually seen in cerebrospinal meningitis
treated by other methods.

The three principal effects of the use of the serum seem to be:
First, to produce a fall of temperature; second, to produce a
rapid improvement in the patient's general condition, accompanied
by a more or less marked relief of certain symptoms; and, third,
to cut short the course of the disease.

The most striking effect on the temperature is a permanent
critical fall following the first dose of serum. Other cases showed
a similar critical fall of temperature, which was, however, not
permanent, the temperature rising again and finally coming down
by lysis. Another effect was seen in a rapid permanent lysis,
which was very striking in cases in which there had been a consistent high temperature up to the time when the first dose of
serum was given. In other cases temporary relapses occurred,
and in some there was no immediate effect.

The effect on the symptoms and general condition is the most
striking phenomenon observed with the use of the serum. In some
cases there occurred a permanent return to consciousness, a disappearance of mental dullness, a disappearance of delirium, and
a disappearance of headache, hyperesthesia, tenderness of the
neck or vomiting. These symptoms were often relieved completely within twenty-four hours after the first injection, the patient
changing in the most remarkable way from a serious condition
of coma to a favorable condition of normal mental activity.

At other times the improvement in this set of symptoms
occurred more slowly, and at still other times, particularly in the
late chronic cases, no such effect was noted.

As to the cutting short of the disease, the average length of
time which patients remained under treatment was but a small
fraction of the time which patients who recovered, remained under
treatment at the hospital in previous years.

Another notable effect of the serum is seen in the successive
examinations of the cerebrospinal fluid during the period of its
use. This effect is most striking in early cases, in which the cerebrospinal fluid contains large numbers of diplococci. In such a
case a great many intracellular diplococci are observed in the
fluid withdrawn by the first lumbar puncture. Twenty-four hours

after the first injection the fluid presents a strikingly different picture. The whole number of organisms seen is much smaller, but the chief change is that the majority are intracellular, only rare extracellular forms being seen. The third lumbar puncture shows still fewer diplococci, and those only intracellular. In the fourth fluid, after three doses, there are frequently no diplococci to be found, or, at most, very rare intracellular forms.

Relapses sometimes occur under the use of the serum. In a relapse, after a period of improvement, the symptoms begin to recur and the temperature to rise. These relapses usually yielded to repeated doses of antiserum.

The completeness of recovery is another noteworthy point in this series. There were sequelæ in 2 cases only, one child being deaf and one blind and deaf.

The results of the use of the serum appeared to depend chiefly on how early it was first used. The earlier it was employed the more marked were its effects.

We may conclude that the prospects of aborting or rapidly cutting short epidemic cerebrospinal meningitis are better the earlier in the disease the serum is given, and that the antiserum usually has no effect in the late chronic stage. There were cases which proved exceptions to this rule, as in 3 cases in which the serum was used comparatively early the patients died. On the other hand, one patient in the late chronic stage began to improve immediately after one dose of serum and made a rapid convalescence. This would show that there is always some hope of a good result so long as diplococci are present. I believe the serum in most cases causes a cessation of the active process and that the resulting course of the disease depends mainly on the extent of tissue damage which has already been done.

As to the amount of serum which should be given, I believe that 30 c.c. can be given usually with perfect safety, even when smaller amounts of fluid are withdrawn. I have given, without any bad results, as much as this when no fluid was withdrawn. One can judge to a certain extent how far it is safe to go by the feeling of resistance to the injection of the serum. In cases in which larger amounts of fluid are withdrawn I believe 45 c.c. should be given at a dose.

The daily injection of the serum in most cases seemed to be effective. After four doses have been given, if, after one or two days the case proves resistant, or at any time if there is a tendency to relapse, this treatment should be repeated. It is a question whether in some severe cases the serum should not be administered oftener than once in twenty-four hours.

I conclude from this series that:—

(1)   The use of the Flexner antiserum is of great value in epidemic cerebrospinal meningitis. I believe its value to be comparable to that of diphtheria antitoxin in diphtheria.

(2)   The use of the serum at times aborts the disease, frequently rapidly relieves its symptoms, shortens its course, lessens the liability to sequelæ, and greatly reduces its mortality.

(3)   The serum should be used as early as possible in all cases, even of suspected epidemic meningitis.

(4)   It should be frequently repeated as long as there are symptoms or any tendency to relapse.

(5)   Late chronic cases are unfavorable for the use of the serum, but any case in which the diplococci are present has some hope of relief by its use.

(6)   Some cases are resistant.

HYDROCEPHALUS OF MENINGOCOCCUS ORIGIN, WITH A SUMMARY OF RECENT CASES OF MENINGITIS TREATED BY ANTIMENINGOCOCCUS SERUM.

BY J. H. MASON KNOX, JR., PH.D., M.D.,

Instructor in Pediatrics in the Johns Hopkins Medical School.

AND

FRANK J. SLADEN, M.D.,

Assistant in Medicine in the Johns Hopkins Medical School.

Introductory.—An increase in the cerebrospinal fluid in inflammation of the meninges has been recognized for many years. Judging, however, from the comparatively small number of cases reported, the definite association of hydrocephalus with cerebrospinal meningitis has not attracted wide attention. This is in part explained by the insidious onset which frequently characterizes hydrocephalus, masking its connection with an antecedent attack of meningitis. Moreover, an increase in intraventricular fluid when of moderate degree in an adult skull, which admits of no dilatation, produces a rather vague and uncertain train of symptoms and may so escape detection. However, in nearly all the text-books, cerebrospinal meningitis is set down among the several causes suggested for the remarkable condition, hydrocephalus, the pathology of which is still so unsettled.

Historical.—Joslin,[1] in a partial review of the history of internal hydrocephalus following cerebrospinal fever, finds that in the same year, 1805, in which epidemic cerebrospinal meningitis is considered to have appeared, a case occurred in Strasburg having typical symptoms, and which on autopsy besides the meningeal congestion and inflammation showed the ventricles to be dilated with turbid serum.

A good description of this complication appears in Foerster's text-book of "Pathological Anatomy,"[2] published in 1863. Two years later, Ziemsen and Hess[3] especially directed attention to hydrocephalus during an epidemic of cerebrospinal meningitis in Erlange. They reported 4 cases with autopsies. Several additional

instances have been published, among others, by Merkel,[4] Niemeyer,[5] Bohmer,[6] Bonsaing,[7] Pimser,[8] Collins,[9] Hart,[10] and von
Hartung.[11] The clinical symptoms and the pathological findings
of the reported cases show striking similarity. After the acute
symptoms of onset there may be marked improvement, which
continues indefinitely, or may be interrupted by paroxysms of
severe headache, pain in neck and extremities, vomiting, loss of
consciousness or convulsions; often there is fever. These
symptoms may subside and remain absent for long periods, during
which the patient may appear quite well, although abnormalities
in the power of concentration or in reflex reaction are usually
present. In a number of cases there is no period of convalescence,
the symptoms attributable to the hydrocephalus following immediately after those of the meningitis.

According to Ziemsen,[12] to whose description of the anatomical findings in 1874 little has been added, after the second or
third week the meningeal exudate begins to break down and to be
absorbed, and there is an increase in the connective tissue of the
serous membranes. The hyperemia of the brain, which marks
the acute stage, subsides. At the same time, usually in about the
fifth to eighth week, the exudate in the ventricles becomes
purulent. Still later there is hyperplasia of the ependyma, then
often fibrous thickening. The ventricular exudate increases in
amount, becomes clearer, the cellular contents tend to sink to the
posterior horns. In many cases there is definite edema of the
brain substance. The choroid plexus becomes blanched. The
brain tissue softens, is continually pressed upon by the increasing fluid and gradually atrophies—it may be to a mere shell.
Most of the cases prove fatal before these advanced changes take
place. The inflammation appears to be carried to the ventricular
ependyma along the course of the blood vessels, extending into
the brain substance from the meninges. Merkel (loc. cit.)
found an extensive cellular proliferation about the vessels of the
ependyma and plexus. It is probable, too, that a venous stasis
is partly brought about by increased intraventricular pressure,
and so further infiltration of fluid is encouraged.

Hulsmann,[13] who makes this condition the subject of his
inaugural dissertation, reports a remarkable case, which shows
how extensive the cerebral alterations may be without symptoms.
The patient was a child of three years, who was suddenly seized

with the symptoms of cerebrospinal meningitis. There was well marked opisthotonus, violent vomiting and fever. After a short period of improvement, convulsive attacks set in and returned at frequent intervals. The patient lost weight rapidly, and after three and one-half months was greatly wasted and showed signs of mental impairment. The sight became completely lost. From this condition the boy gradually improved, and in another month had, to all appearances, recovered complete health. The eyesight returned completely, and the mother considered the patient the brightest of her several children. After eight months of perfect health the child, together with several other members of the family, died of diphtheria. On autopsy, a pronounced hydro-cephalus was found. All the ventricles were dilated, and there was well-marked granulation and thickening of the ependymal lining—evidently the result of the previous meningitis.

An apparently identical condition in an infant is also re-ported by Grosz[14] in 1899. The patient, a boy of ten months, was brought to the hospital with the history of having been seized six weeks before with fever and repeated convulsions. The head was retracted. A month later the symptoms subsided, but the eyes were crossed and five days before admission became blind. On examination the head was found to be large, the sagittal sutures open and the anterior fontanel bulging. The pupils did not react to light or accommodation; the eye grounds were normal. There was slight light perception. Evidently an internal hydrocephalus had followed the meningitis and the blindness resulted from increased intracranial pressure. Through a ventricular puncture, 40 c.c. of clear fluid were removed, which was followed at once by an improvement in the child's general condition. The eyes became less crossed. At a second puncture, a few days later, 70 c.c. of fluid were removed. Convalescence afterward was uninterrupted and the child's condition was re-ported excellent eleven months after leaving the hospital.

Dr. Osler,[15] under the title, "Chronic Meningitis," and, lately, Cuno,[16] of Frankfort, report somewhat similar cases.

Cases in which permanent mental impairment has followed the development of internal hydrocephalus after meningitis have been reported by Heubner,[17] Hulsmann,[18] and many others.

Holt,[18] in 1887, published an instance of chronic hydro-cephalus in a child of thirteen months. The enlargement of the

head had been noticed at three months, and the patient's development had been much retarded. On section marked pachymenin-
gitis was found over the whole brain. The ventricles were much
dilated. There were no signs of acute inflammation and no
history pointing definitely to cerebrospinal fever.

In the exhaustive treatise of Councilman, Mallory and
Wright[19] on "Epidemic Cerebrospinal Meningitis in 1898," little
mention is made of hydrocephalus, but in the autopsy records
of 35 cases the lateral ventricles were found to be dilated in at
least 5 instances, and in 5 others the exudation at the base was
described as abundant. In a majority of these cases, the
ependymal lining of the ventricles was shown to be granular.

Wentworth[20] in the same year, when an extensive epidemic
of cerebrospinal fever occurred in Boston, did not refer specifically to cases of hydrocephalus in infants as a consequence, but
did report a case of chronic meningitis with autopsy, in which
the ventricles were dilated. The condition was not especially
associated with meningitis by Koplik,[21] who described the clinical
features of the many cases coming under his observation in the
New York epidemic of 1903 and 1904.

In the "Reports of St. Thomas Hospital, London," for 1899,[22]
an instance of acute hydrocephalus following typical meningitis
is described in a man aged thirty. The illness was of but five
weeks' duration. On autopsy the ventricles were found to be
dilated and the membranes opaque and thickened.

A year later Joslin,[1] of Boston, reported 8 similar cases in
patients between sixteen and thirty-two years of age. There
seems to have been no special association between the severity
of the meningitis and the development of the hydrocephalus. In
several instances a number of weeks elapsed between the termination of all signs of meningitis and the onset of symptoms referable to hydrocephalus. There were headache, vomiting, restlessness, occasional delirium and convulsions. Strabismus and a return of fever were often noted. On autopsy, in all of these cases,
in addition to the dilatation of the ventricles, the ependymal
lining was found to be swollen and granular and floor of the
fourth ventricle thickened. In the horns of the lateral ventricles
were collections of fibrin-like flakes. The pia mater was much
thickened, especially along the course of the blood vessels. In
several of the cases cultures were taken from the ventricular fluid
and were found to be sterile.

A case somewhat similar to those we shall here report was seen by Northrup[28] in 1896. It concerned a boy of three years, who ran a course of what was clinically cerebrospinal fever. After four months he seemed to have completely recovered, but died six months from the onset of illness. On autopsy the convolutions of the brain were found to be much flattened and the ventricular fluid four times the normal amount. The ependyma were granular. There was no evidence anywhere of tuberculosis.

Our attention has been directed to this increase in the intracranial pressure as a result of cerebrospinal fever due to infection with the meningococcus by the two following cases:—

CASE I. A baby aged five months, was seen in consultation on November 7th last year. The family history was unimportant. The birth had been normal and the child had flourished for two months at the breast. At this time it was weaned and there had been some indigestion on artificial feeding, with little gain afterward.

The present illness began seven weeks before, when the baby, without warning, was seized with a general convulsion, followed by vomiting and fever. These symptoms abated and after two weeks the child seemed to be becoming better when the fever returned and the stiffness of the neck was noticed. Since this time there had been a continuous irregular fever and occasional convulsions, which were becoming more frequent. There was also frequent vomiting, although the stools were normal. When seen, the baby was lying with head much retracted. The head was large, being about 44 cm. in circumference. The anterior fontanel was tense and bulging and the bones of the head unduly separated by intracranial pressure. The pupils were contracted and reacted sluggishly to light. The chest was clear; the heart action was markedly irregular. The abdomen was negative, the skin evidently hypersensitive to pressure. Kernig's sign was positive. It was, of course, clear that the child had meningitis, and that many of the alarming symptoms were due to increased cerebral pressure. Lumbar puncture was immediately performed, and 100 c.c. of slightly turbid fluid under high tension was withdrawn. This fluid was found to contain many pus cells and a small number of intracellular diplococci. The use of the Flexner serum was suggested, but declined. It was not urged, because it was then felt that in cases of such long standing it would be of little service. For several days afterward the symptoms abated, but on November 13th, a week later, it was necessary to repeat the puncture; 100 c.c. of fluid of the same character was removed. The patient was seen by us on these two occasions only. For several weeks from this time the child was said to be better. He took nourishment well, was in less pain and the convulsions had almost ceased. The retraction of the neck, however, persisted. Late in December the father said the baby was much improved and asked about engaging a nursery maid. A few days later the child died suddenly, four months after the onset of symptoms. No autopsy was obtained. Diagnosis: Acute, then chronic, cerebrospinal meningitis of meningococcus origin; acute internal hydrocephalus.

CASE II. In March of this year one of us was asked by a nurse at the milk dispensaries to see a child in South Baltimore, who had recently begun taking milk at the station, and who appeared very ill. The patient, a boy of six months, was found lying on a pillow. The size of the head at once attracted attention. It was considerably enlarged and had to be supported. The baby was much emaciated and very fretful. The history at that time was most indefinite. No reason for this condition could be assigned by the parents. The mother had first noticed the enlarged head about five weeks before. The left side of the head bulged out distinctly more than the right; the scalp on the left side seemed a trifle reddened. The baby's birth was said to have been normal. It had been breast-fed for two months, afterward it was fed, for the most part, on cow's milk. There had been constant indigestion; there was no stigmata of rickets.

The anterior fontanel was large and tense and the bones of the head widely separated. It was not clear just what the condition was which was responsible for increase in the intracranial pressure. A neoplasm was suspected. The parents were persuaded to come to the dispensary, where a consultation was obtained with Dr. Cushing. Dr. Cushing did a lumbar puncture, but obtained only a few drops of serous fluid. He then punctured the ventricle and removed 120 c.c. of straw-colored fluid. A crinoline bandage was applied and the child sent home with the diagnosis of chronic internal hydrocephalus, probably of congenital origin, the thought being that the parents had not detected the early enlargement of the head.

When the fluid from the ventricle was examined by Dr. Sladen, it was found to contain many extra and intracellular diplococci, which on culture proved to be the diplococci of Weichelbaum. The patient was sent for and admitted to Dr. Barker's service on March 21, 1908, that he might be treated with the antimeningococcus serum. In the ward, on close questioning, it was discovered that four months before, at the age of two months, the child had once waked from sleep moaning, evidently suffering great pain. One hour afterward it had a general clonic convulsion lasting two minutes, followed by several others less severe the next day. For the following four days and nights the child cried constantly. The eyes were crossed, and he was feverish. The only other convulsion occurred three weeks after this onset. During the last three months the patient had constantly lost in weight. The increase in the size of the head began five weeks before admission. He had been treated in his home for pneumonia, muscular rheumatism, indigestion and intestinal rickets.

On admission, the child was found to be as already described, an extremely emaciated baby. Both fontanels bulged and the head sutures were gaping. Circumference, 46.5 cm. The pupils were wide and reacted to light. The head was somewhat retracted and the neck held stiffly. The back was not arched. The chest and abdomen presented no abnormalities. The knee kicks were not obtained. Kernig's sign was not positive in either side. The leukocytes numbered 17,000.

By a second lumbar puncture about 2 c.c. of a blood-stained fluid were obtained. This was sterile. The child was put on a milk and oatmeal water diet and given a hot bath and a cocoa butter rub every day. His general condition improved after admission until just before the final collapse. He took nourishment greedily, slept soundly and gained 250 grams in fourteen days in spite of several ventricular punctures. Examination of the eyes by Dr. Bordley disclosed double choked disk, the one near the papillæ being large and tortuous. Fluid was removed by tapping the ventricle on four additional occasions, five in all, March 28th, 31st, April 3d and 8th, at which times 150 c.c., 100 c.c., 60 c.c. and 140 c.c., respectively, were taken. Antimeningitis serum (Flexner) was given immediately after four of the tappings, each time 15 c.c. were injected, the first time into the lumbar meninges, the other times into the ventricle. None of the taps seemed to disturb the patient very much. There was no collapse. The meningococci were found each time in the cerebral fluid, but seemed fewer in the fluid last removed. The child ran an irregular temperature, ranging from 96.4° to 101.8°. The respiration varied from 24 to 40, the pulse from 100 to 50.

Early in the morning of April 8th, when symptoms seemed favorable, the patient suddenly went into collapse; Cheyne-Stokes' breathing developed, due apparently to a sudden increase in intraventricular pressure. A ventricular tap was done four hours later, but the patient did not rally and died at noon. No autopsy was allowed.

These cases are reported because the number of similar instances in which the causal organisms have been found in the hydrocephalic fluid are certainly few. The symptoms of the condition have been dwelt upon sufficiently in recounting the cases. The length of time the meningococci remained viable in the ventricular fluid from the onset of symptoms is noteworthy, and suggests that similar findings may be true of some of the cases thought to be idiopathic hydrocephalus.

The uncertainty of the outcome has recently been emphasized by Huber.[24] As regards the prevention or cure of the condition there is much of encouragement in the results obtained in the treatment of cerebrospinal meningitis by the specific antiserum. Unquestionably the inflammatory process produced by the meningococcus causes the initial reaction in the ependymal lining leading to increased exudation of fluid. When this is present in excess it may readily tend to produce venous stasis, and so further increase the condition. If the serum treatment provides an efficient opponent to the action of the specific microorganism, the number of cases of meningitis that advance to the stage of hydrocephalus should be further lessened, and, moreover, the condition itself, when due, as it was in the last case cited, to viable cocci, should yield to intraventricular injection. The immediate effects of cerebral hypertension can be, to a large extent, avoided by occasional lumbar or ventricular puncture.

Through the courtesy of Dr. Barker, in addition to the foregoing case, we are permitted to present a summary of the cases of meningococcus cerebrospinal meningitis treated by an antimeningitis serum (Flexner) in the wards of the Johns Hopkins Hospital during the past year. Two of these cases were seen by one of us before they entered the hospital and will be referred to briefly. The first concerns a boy, white, aged fifteen years, seen with Dr. H. L. Whittle, of Baltimore. His family and personal history were good. There had been few previous illnesses. The patient had complained eighteen days before of chilly sensations and pains in the limbs. At that time he had a cold, coryza and cough with expectoration. His appetite was impaired, and he felt ill, but continued at work, that of a clerk. Sixteen days later he was obliged to stop work on account of a severe frontal headache. He complained also of pain in his back, and his temperature arose to 104°, pulse 132, respirations 28. That night he had three clonic convulsions, involving the whole body; the last one was an hour in duration. The rigidity of his head and lips soon became marked. The following afternoon the patient was hypersensitive and cried with pain when his head was moved. Shortly afterward he became somewhat delirious. Occasionally a convergent and divergent strabismus was noted. There was no history of vomiting. At this time an eruption described as red-pinhead spots appeared over the greater part of the chest, abdomen, back and thighs. There were physical signs of bronchitis. When seen the patient was quite unconscious with marked rigidity of neck, retracted pupils, definite Kernig's sign, and intense hyperesthesia. There was no question, whatever, about the diagnosis or the serious character of the ailment, and the patient was removed at once to the hospital in an ambulance. By lumbar puncture under anesthesia at the hospital, cerebrospinal fluid was found to have a pressure of more than 400 mm.; 20 c.c. of this fluid were removed and 14 c.c. of antimeningitis serum were injected. In the following seventy-five days lumbar puncture was performed five times more, and on each occasion was followed by the injection of serum. Numerous meningococci were present. In sixteen days 230 c.c. of cerebrospinal fluid were removed and 150 c.c. of serum given. Temporary improvement followed each injection, but his condition was not permanently bettered until the seventeenth day of his illness. After this time all symptoms subsided, and convalescence ending in complete recovery began.

Treatment besides the serum injection was eliminative and

supporting. This case was evidently one of very severe infection, which we feel confident would have ended fatally, in short order, had it not been for the use of the serum. With this treatment, even, convalescence was long delayed, but the response to the injection of serum seemed definite.

The other instance is that of a child, aged seven years. Thirteen days before seen he came home from school complaining of headache. He went to bed, became feverish, vomited, and that evening was somewhat delirious. He had remained more or less in this condition since. The neck was stiff and his eyes were crossed for nine days. The skin was definitely hypersensitive. On examination he was found to be much emaciated, with the eruption of herpes on the lips. Tongue was coated, the head retracted, the neck markedly stiff, the chest and abdomen negative, excepting that the latter was scaphoid. Kernig's sign was present. Leukocytes were 16,400. He was at once sent to the hospital, where a lumbar puncture was done, and a cloudy fluid removed containing leukocytes and meningococci; 30 c.c. of antimeningitis serum were injected. Some improvement in his condition followed. A second puncture with serum injection was performed on the following day. The fluid removed showed a definite increase in polymorphonuclear leukocytes and a marked diminution in the number of organisms. Convalescence after this time was uninterrupted and the patient was discharged well on the thirty-fifth day of his disease, twenty days after admission. In this instance, it seems that the patient might have recovered without the serum treatment, but unquestionably the convalescence was hastened and the result made more certain because of this procedure.

During the year ending May, 1908, 21 cases of meningitis, shown by bacteriological examination of the cerebrospinal fluid to be due to the meningococcus of Weichselbaum, have been treated with the serum. Three of the 21 cases died, a mortality of 14 per cent. Of 12 cases under the age of twelve years, 1 died, a mortality of 8 per cent.

The effect *first* upon the temperature has been to cause a rapid fall. One case remained normal after a simple injection, but the majority showed a rise the next day and required at least three injections to preserve a normal temperature. As many cases have recovered by crisis as by lysis.

Secondly, with the fall in temperature, in three to twelve

hours, the symptoms and signs began to clear. The symptoms, headache, delirium, pain in the neck and back, and the general hyperesthesis disappeared with remarkable rapidity. The signs, strabismus, stiffness of the neck, and the Kernig sign, were more persistent. The Kernig was often the last sign to disappear. Strangely, pressure signs and symptoms were relieved by the treatment, notwithstanding the fact that the spinal fluid removed was often replaced by the same amount of serum—in several instances by more serum.

Thirdly, the effect upon the spinal fluid itself was striking. The polymorphonuclear leukocytes were increased in the spinal fluid after the first injection, disappearing as the process healed. The cells in 1 case were increased from 200 to the c.mm. to 4,000. The influence of this upon the leukocytes in the circulating blood is quite evident. The white cells in the circulation are decreased by the increased demand for them in the spinal fluid. In every case there is a very constant, positive chemiotaxis for polymorphonuclear leukocytes in the spinal fluid.

In 6 cases of tuberculous meningitis the clear fluid with predominating small mononuclear cells became clouded with polymorphonuclears, and the small mononuclears entirely disappeared. The increase in cells was observed in a case of influenzal meningitis, but the serum caused no evident change in 2 cases of pneumococcal meningitis.

The meningococci mainly extracellular at first become intracellular after serum. Phagocytosis is promoted, so that it is difficult to find organisms outside of cells in specimens after serum.

The diplococci besides becoming intracellular are evidently being destroyed. They no longer stain deeply and distinctly, but are ill-defined and hard to see. This is evidenced by the cultures. The first specimens give an abundant growth. But after serum, the same amount of centrifugalized sediment will give from two to ten colonies, and many cultures have remained sterile after a single injection.

Although it is bold to venture to characterize the serum when Dr. Flexner himself will not do so, still, clinically, we are impressed with the rapid disappearance of signs and symptoms, which speaks for an antitoxic power. The positive chemiotaxis for polymorphonuclear leukocytes and the promoted phagocytosis are

the most constant features.   And finally the reduction in the
number of diplococci, the change in staining properties, and the
loss of viability, speak for a bactericidal power—though this may
be explained by the phagocytosis.

　　We acknowledge with pleasure our indebtedness to Dr. L. F.
Barker for allowing us to make use of the cases in his wards.

REFERENCES.

1.　Joslin.　American Journal of Medical Science, 1900, Vol. CXX., p. 444.
2.　Foerster.　Pathological Anatomy, 1863, p. 597.
3.　Ziemsen and Hess.　Deut. Ach. für Klin. Med., Vol. I.
4.　Merkel.　Ibid.
5.　Niemeyer.　Die Epidem. Cerebrospinal Meningitis, etc., Berlin, 1865.
6.　Bohmer.　Bayr Arztl Intelligenz., 1865, p. 39.
7.　Bonsaing.　Wiener Med. Presse, 1868, p. 19.
8.　Pimser.　Wien. Med. Woch., pp. 30, 33, 51, 52.
9.　Collins.　Dublin Quarterly Journal, 1868, XLVI., p. 170.
10.　Hart.　St. Bartholomew's Hospital Reports, 1876.
11.　von Hartung.　Ueber Epidem. Cerebrospinal Meningitis, Inaug. Disc. Kiel, 1888.
12.　Ziemsen.　Handbuch d. Acuten Infect. Krank., 1874, p. 683.
13.　Hulsmann.　Drei Falle von Chroneschem Hydrocephalus nach abyelaufener Meningitis Cerebrospinal Epidemica, Inaug. Disc. Kiel, 1889.
14.　Groez.　Archiv. für Kinderhk., 1899, Vol. XXVII., p. 285.
15.　Osler.　The Johns Hopkins Hospital Bulletin, 1892, 118.
16.　Cuno.　Abs. Centralb. für Kinderhk., 1906, Vol. XI., p. 152.
17.　Heubner.　Eulenberg's Encyclopedia, 3d ed., p. 430.
18.　Holt.　ARCHIVES OF PEDIATRICS, 1887, Vol. IV., p. 741.
19.　Councilman, Mallory and Wright.　Epidemic Cerebrospinal Meningitis, Boston, 1898.
20.　Wentworth.　Boston Medical and Surgical Journal, 1898, Vol. CXXXVIII., p. 270.
21.　Koplik.　New York Medical News, 1904, Vol. LXXXIV., p. 1,065.
22.　St. Thomas' Hospital Reports, 1899. p. 65.
23.　Northrup.　ARCHIVES OF PEDIATRICS, 1896, Vol. XIII., p. 901.
24.　Huber.　ARCHIVES OF PEDIATRICS, 1908, Vol. XXII., p. 80.

THE DIAGNOSTIC VALUE OF THE CHEMICAL AND BACTERIOLOGICAL EXAMINATION OF CEREBROSPINAL FLUID.

BY ALFRED HAND, JR., M.D.,

Philadelphia.

The exact diagnosis of the different forms of meningitis is always important. With the introduction of a specific treatment for one of the forms, which as Pepper used to say "maims for life when it does not kill, as does no other disease, save possibly scarlet fever," the importance is greatly increased of arriving at an exact diagnosis as early as possible. Thanks to Quincke, lumbar puncture furnishes the means of making an exact diagnosis. But the fluid obtained by lumbar puncture must always be examined with great care in order to arrive at a correct interpretation. There may be said to be two main types of cerebrospinal fluid, one in which the interpretation is easy and the other in which it is difficult. It is easy when the fluid is typical of one or another form of meningitis, but in the majority of cases it requires a painstaking, careful examination. Typical specimens present well-marked contrasts. Thus, if the fluid from a case of meningitis shows a milky opalescence, which disappears as the fibrin-network forms, leaving a clear fluid which contains a great increase in the normal amount of albumin and with the presence of sugar but little if any below the normal percentage, the fibrin network also being found to contain mainly mononuclear leukocytes and tubercle bacilli, the diagnosis is clearly tuberculous meningitis. If the fluid is distinctly turbid, with sometimes a slight yellowish tint, and polynuclear leukocytes are found in abundance some of them containing in their protoplasm diplococci, the diagnosis is established of epidemic cerebrospinal fever; after the fibrin network has formed and been withdrawn, further study of the fluid will show moderate increase in the albumin and total absence of sugar. A pneumococcic meningitis gives a very similar fluid, with occasionally a greenish-yellow tint, as in strepto- or staphylococcic meningitis, but the diplococcus in this form is hardly ever

seen in the pus cells, being very abundant in the fluid. (In the two
latest cases of pneumococcic meningitis which I have seen, the
fluid from one secondary to an otitis had a few leukocytes which
contained diplococci, while the majority of the germs were free
in the fluid, and the fluid from the other, secondary to a small
pneumonic focus, showed every polynuclear leukocyte surrounded
by a complete ring of diplococci but none in the protoplasm). The
fluid in this and other septic forms resembles that in the epidemic
form in having a moderate increase in albumin and a total absence
of sugar.

But the fluid obtained by lumbar puncture may not have these
striking characteristics; it may be only slightly turbid or apparently perfectly clear, so that it is well to have a systematic method
of examination. The first step of importance is to start the examination as soon after the fluid is obtained as possible. It is well
to allow a drop to fall from the needle on to a slide; or shortly
after collecting the fluid, a loopful is transferred to a slide, evaporated, and the film stained immediately. The meningococcus may
then be found in great numbers in some cases, while an examination postponed over night may fail to show any germs whatever.
Having taken this film and also cultures, which may also be made
while the fluid is flowing from the needle, or soon after, the test
tube containing the fluid is allowed to stand for several hours in
order that the leukocytes and bacteria may sink and the fibrin-
network form. Then with a straight platinum needle the network
is carefully transferred to a slide, the best preparation being obtained by tilting the test tube so that the fibrin always floats in the
fluid. It is then possible to spread out the network on the slide,
evaporate the fluid and fix by heat. Before staining this preparation, it will save time to conduct a chemical examination of the
fluid. Half of it may be used for a quantitative estimation of the
albumin, and for this purpose the acetic acid and potassium fer-
rocyanid test in the graduated urine tubes and the centrifuge is
convenient and seems to me to be reasonably accurate. At least,
I have always found a fairly constant result for the different
forms of meningitis. This test gives the bulk percentage of albumin, and every specimen of tuberculous meningitis I have examined has shown 5 per cent. or over, the usual amount being
about 9 per cent. or 10 per cent. The other forms of meningitis
have never exceeded 5 per cent. in my experience, the average

being 3 per cent. or 4 per cent., the amount in normal fluid being one-half of 1 per cent.

The other half of the fluid should be used for the phenylhydrazin test for sugar; Fehling's solution may be used, but there is often not enough fluid to give a reaction, and the phenylhydrazin test is much more delicate.

The results of these two tests will serve as a guide for staining the slide previously prepared. If the albumin is above 5 per cent. by bulk and if sugar is present, then the staining should be for tubercle bacilli, with a mechanical stage used for the search, which will be rewarded with a positive result in something over 99 per cent. if the technic has been carefully followed.

If the albumin is below 5 per cent. and sugar is absent, it is hardly worth while to stain for tubercle bacilli, but the examination may then be devoted to a search for the meningococcus. It is sometimes impossible to decide whether a case is of the epidemic or pneumococcic variety, as the slide may show only a few isolated cocci, or even none at all.

I have thus far laid little stress on a differential count of the leukocytes; this is often of great value, when it can be made, but the cells are often distorted or degenerated and it is difficult in some cases to decide their true form.

The fact that the tuberculous form is associated with the persistence of sugar in the fluid and the almost total absence of polynuclear leukocytes, while the reverse holds for other infections led me to think that perhaps there was some relation between the two and that inasmuch as a proteolytic ferment has been obtained from degenerating leukocytes there might perhaps be also a sugar-splitting ferment. The experiments which I made are incomplete as yet, owing to a lack of coincidence of suitable material, but a preliminary report follows.

Pus from an empyema was used, giving no reduction of Fehling's solution.

One drop of pus from each c.c. was added to a 0.5 per cent. solution of glucose, giving a fluid of about the degree of turbidity of a pneumococcic meningitis, and the mixture was incubated for twenty-four hours at 37.5° C; at the end of that time the sugar was reduced exactly one-half, to 0.25 per cent.

Cultures of the pus on agar and blood-serum gave staphylococci. Another tube containing 0.5 per cent. glucose solution was inoculated with the germs and incubated for thirty-two hours, with an almost imperceptible lessening in the amount of sugar, the resulting calculation giving 0.49 per cent.

These results, if confirmed by subsequent tests, point to the existence of a sugar-splitting ferment in polynuclear leukocytes.

(Since writing the above, I have had an opportunity to use Flexner's antiserum in a case of meningococcic meningitis, the resulting changes in the characteristics of the fluid being extremely interesting. At the first tapping 45 c.c. of turbid fluid literally spouted from the needle; sugar was absent, albumin was increased to 5 per cent. by bulk, many leukocytes were present, staining very poorly with the outlines of the cells and nuclei very indistinct, a few of them containing diplococci. Injections of antiserum were given on the three days following, the fluid at the second and third tappings resembling that at the first, with 45 c.c. each time; at the fourth tapping, when the last dose of antiserum was given, only 15 c.c. were obtained, the albumin being slightly increased to 6 per cent., the leukocytes being well-preserved, polynuclears being in the majority but mononuclears being abundant, a few diplococci being found; and sugar was also present, probably an indication of a return to the normal condition of the fluid, as no further tappings were necessary, recovery being speedy).

THE SERUM TREATMENT AND THE PROGNOSIS, UNDER VARIOUS FORMS OF THERAPY, OF CEREBROSPINAL FEVER.

BY HENRY KOPLIK, M.D.,

New York.

It is too often apparent in considering the methods of therapy of any disease that we sometimes lose sight in the presence of some exceedingly favorable results of the natural course of the affection, and in no disease is this more common than in cerebrospinal meningitis. This disease, as Osler has pointed out, resembles very closely in its behavior pneumonia. It is true the affection occurs sporadically and in epidemics. In the sporadic form the disease occurs at times when there cannot be said to be any prevalent epidemic. That is, a limited number of cases will appear in a city in places removed from each other, and having no connection with each other. By epidemics of meningitis we understand distinctly the occurrence in larger numbers of cases in groups, and in this disease, especially in densely populated quarters. In the sporadic form cerebrospinal fever is an affection at times so mild as to give few symptoms of a critical nature. At other times in the sporadic form the disease takes on a severer type, and then the picture closely resembles what is seen in epidemics of the disease. In the absence of epidemics the cases of cerebrospinal meningitis which have come under our control have impressed us with certain characteristics, or, rather, the absence of certain characteristics which we see during the times of epidemics. I have seen sporadic cases so mild that the intermittent or remittent febrile symptoms, headache and drowsiness, were the only symptoms which led us to think of the diagnosis. In the sporadic forms we have the rigidity, the hyperesthesia, the presence of the Kernig reaction, and in occasional cases the herpes. There is also delirium and the presence of gradually increasing hydrocephalus, as evinced by the so-called Macewen sign. I think any one who has passed through an epidemic of cerebrospinal meningitis will admit that in the sporadic cases we rarely meet the severer symptoms of the disease, such as the sudden and abrupt onset of unconsciousness, the petechiæ or diffuse hemorrhages so frequent in the epidemic forms of the disease, and the paralysis which appears very early in the epidemic forms. In fact, in an epidemic it is not infrequent to be called to the bedside to see a child who within a few hours has become unconscious and absolutely paretic to an extent as not even to show the rigidity and the Kernig sign, which is seen and gradually develops so classically in the sporadic cases. In the sporadic cases we rarely see those excessive hemorrhages in infants which are seen in the epidemic form.

It must, therefore, be admitted that though on the whole the symptomatology of the sporadic is exactly similar to that of the epidemic form of the disease, the sporadic form runs a much milder course. As we analyze both forms more deeply, we find that the purulent exudates are more frequently obtained in the epidemic than in the sporadic cases of the disease. Lumbar puncture in the sporadic cases exceptionally reveals a purulent fluid at the outset. It is true a certain proportion of the sporadic cases are purulent, but not to the extent as is seen in the epidemic forms of the disease.

In a word, cerebrospinal meningitis of the meningococcic type very much resembles pneumonia as it is seen in adults in the sporadic and epidemic forms. Any one who has lived through an epidemic of pneumonia must admit that the picture is a violent and a virulent one in its type, and so with meningitis. We have the same infection, but in the epidemic form it is of a violent and virulent type, and with children the younger the subject the more fatal the disease.

These facts are so self-evident that it is surprising they are so constantly lost sight of, and that in considering any mode of therapy we do not stop not only to consider the violence of the infection, but the age of the patient. For this reason I have thought it would be useful for every one at this time to get a picture of the natural history and prognosis of cerebrospinal meningitis, especially if the experience which reflects the prognosis extends over a long period of time and the methods of treatment have been uniformly the same and carefully carried out in all details through a number of years.

Taking up the sporadic form of meningococcic cerebrospinal

meningitis, I have been fortunate to have at my disposal the records of cases treated since 1899 up to the epidemic years of 1904-1905. We first began the systematic treatment of cerebrospinal meningitis in 1899. This consisted in the first place of a careful study of the symptoms and the performance of lumbar puncture repeated as often as we found the symptoms to warrant it. That is, a patient suffering with cerebrospinal meningitis would come in with mild symptoms. If there was delirium, high fever, with the development of the signs of fluid in the ventricle as evinced by the Macewen sign, lumbar puncture was performed. After such a puncture, if the symptoms did not abate, the fever continued, as well as the delirium and the Macewen sign persisted, proving that there was a continued hydrocephalus, the patient was again punctured. In this way some patients were punctured two, three, four, and five times, as necessity called for. During 1899-1900 we had 8 cases, all proving by lumbar puncture to have been meningococcic in type. During 1901, 1902 and 1903 there were 13 cases, thus giving us a total of 21 sporadic cases. Of these sporadic cases 8 died, a mortality of 38 per cent.; of these 8 which proved fatal, 6 were below one year of age, thus showing that in the sporadic form the disease was most fatal among the infants below one year of age, and equally so below two years of age. If we could deduct from the total number of 21 cases those which were below one year of age, we would have 15 cases, with only two deaths, a mortality of 13 per cent. From this a mere glance will tell us that meningitis of the meningococcic type in its sporadic form is a comparatively mild disease.

I say this with a certain amount of confidence, although the number of cases is limited, for we are now having a certain number of sporadic cases which seem to duplicate our experience in these years. On the other hand, in sporadic meningitis we have been fortunate by methods of therapy, which consisted mainly in the systematic application of lumbar puncture repeated at intervals, in obtaining recoveries even below one year of age. Two infants of this tender age recovered of these 21 cases, and 2 recovered between the ages of one and two years. It is in the sporadic cases especially that we occasionally see after one lumbar puncture the temperature drop and convalescence practically inaugurated, the temperature not rising subsequently to any extent. This phenomenon is not so frequent nor so persistent as is seen under the new method of therapy, that of serum. Under serum therapy there are more cases which act in this manner than under previous forms of therapy.

Taking up the epidemic years of 1904 and 1905, the history of the disease is a more violent one. Among the cases are some which died within a few hours after admission to the hospital. This, it is understood, is the exception in the sporadic cases, but not uncommon in epidemic cases. Here the picture of the disease is more of sthenic type, the symptoms being developed in their most florid form.

The first epidemic year was 1904. There were 39 cases and 21 deaths, a total mortality of 53 per cent., and of these 21 deaths 13 were below two years of age. If we consider the unimproved cases of these 13 as not fatal, 11 died, but I would prefer to consider these fatal cases as they were discharged from the hospital in a marantic condition, with an incurable and increasing hydrocephalus, so that from a curative standpoint the mortality was practically 100 per cent. Some of these infants were four months of age, some six months of age, showing the tender age of the patients. Deducting these 13 cases from the total of 39 would leave 26 cases above two years of age, of which 9 died, a mortality of 34 per cent.

In 1905 there were 35 cases in my service, of which 17 died. In none of these cases have we included any which have not been distinctly proven by lumbar puncture to be of the meningococcic type. There was thus in this year a total mortality of 48 per cent. Of these 17 deaths, however, 10 were below two years of age, and in them it might be said that the mortality was fully 100 per cent., for if seven died and three were simply unimproved, that is, developed either hydrocephalus or marasmus of an extreme type hopelessly incurable, we can scarcely speak of a cure, therefore these three were no better than fatal cases, so that although there was a mortality of 70 per cent., from the standpoint of success in therapy, the mortality was practically 100 per cent. below two years of age. If we deduct those cases which died below two years of age from the total mortality of 17, and from the total number of cases which were admitted during this epidemic year, we are left a mortality of 7 deaths in 25 cases; that is, 28 per cent. It is thus seen that it would be quite unfair to consider any mortality in this year of the violent type without considering the tender age of some of those affected in order to get a definite idea of the picture. It may be said in addition, the ages of these children ranged from four months to twelve years of age. Thus of the two epidemic years of 1904 and 1905 we had 51 cases above two years of age, with a mortality of 31 per cent., and, considering the patients below two years of age in the mortality, there was a total mortality of 50 per cent. This includes patients on whom there was only an opportunity to make one lumbar puncture, and in whom death occurred within a few hours after admission to the hospital. Nothing has been excluded for the sake of statistics, but the moribund cases have been included in this statistic with the favorable cases. We had 23 cases in these two years below two years of age, of which 78 per cent. died outright, and the remainder were unimproved—that is, those who were discharged with incurable hydrocephalus, idiocy, and marasmus, and which might be considered as practically fatal sooner or later.

From the study of these two sets of statistics one of the sporadic cases of cerebrospinal meningitis and the other of the epidemic form, we see that in the sporadic cases we have succeeded in saving by simple lumbar puncture 4 children below two years of age; in the epidemic cases we have not succeeded in saving any. When I say 4 cases recovered, I mean complete and actual recovery, as far as can be judged from the clinical standpoint. No such cases occurred in the epidemic years. On the other hand, if we deduct from our statistics the cases below two years of age, both in the epidemic and sporadic forms of the disease, we find that in the sporadic form we had 15 cases, with a mortality of 13 per cent., and in the epidemic form we had 51 cases, with a mortality of 31 per cent.

With this history of the disease, we can approach with a certain amount of satisfaction a form of therapy which will hold out an improvement even on these statistics. We can scarcely ask an annullment of mortality. There will always occur cases in either form of the disease which therapy will never reach, no matter how brilliant the conception of the therapy. We see this in diphtheria. No one will deny the great blessing to mankind that the serum treatment of diphtheria has come to be. We have even believed that certain severer forms of diphtheria are becoming less frequent than before the serum therapy. The severer laryngeal types are not so common to-day. even in epidemics of the disease, and this is certainly a great gain. In other words, by the constant application of a form of therapy conceived on a logical basis of antagonism to the bacteria attending the disease, it seems that the actual poison has been diluted and the picture of the disease is a much milder one to-day than before the application of the serum therapy, and thus it may be of other diseases.

Considering cerebrospinal meningitis treated by serum we have to offer 13 cases of the disease occurring in one service, and treated with the exception of the application of the serum, in the identical manner that the cases were treated which have just been spoken of. That is, they were systematically punctured, they were repeatedly punctured, they were punctured only on indications as above detailed in the epidemic and sporadic years, but when punctured they received the serum. They received the serum under conditions exactly similar to those of cases occurring years ago, at a time when the serum did not exist. Our serum cases were thus under the same identical régime as the other cases, and we think that this is of decided advantage not only to the patients, but to others.

It makes quite a difference in the application of such a therapy how such a therapy is applied. A therapy applied by inexperienced hands, no matter how brilliant the therapy, is not given the same chance as in the hands of those who are skillful. We make this remark simply in passing, because any form of therapy will at first labor under a great disadvantage for lack of skillful application and method.

It may not be amiss here to outline very briefly our method of giving the serum to patients. No patient is punctured in my service in cerebrospinal meningitis unless there is distinct indication for that puncture. In this way I impress those around me that I do not believe in the dictum that the earlier the puncture the better. This dictum, I think, is rather mechanical on account of the panicky feeling to do something immediately which it engenders, and does harm to the patient. To be punctured, a patient must show symptoms of pressure and indications of cerebrospinal fluid. There must be not only delirium and sopor, but distinct signs of increase of fluid in the ventricles of the brain, as shown by percussion of the skull. When we get the so-called Macewen percussion note, however slight, in a patient who evinces the symptoms of cerebrospinal meningitis, we proceed to puncture. The puncture is carried out strictly according to Quincke's injunctions. We puncture in the median line in children and adolescents. We withdraw the fluid until we think the pressure is approximately normal in the rachidian space. We then introduce the serum, not with a syringe, but with a funnel. We have found that the funnel as advised by Quincke, a small funnel made of glass capable of holding about 20 c.c., is the best method of introducing the serum, or, for that matter, any fluid into the subarachnoid space, and saves the patient from any accident which might result from the use of a syringe. The pressure exerted by a syringe at all times against the respiratory and vascular pressure is certainly not as gentle a mode of introduction of serum or as safe as allowing the serum to flow into the canal. Thus no traumatism can possibly result, and the fluid finds its way against the negative pressure with the greatest of facility. We repeat the puncture if, after having punctured a patient and introducing the serum, we find that the symptoms do not abate and that the hydrocephalus has either persisted or returns. The temperature is scarcely a guide, but, rather, the general condition of the patient, and especially the presence or absence of hydrocephalus. In this way we think we have made the ideal procedure for the patient.

We have a record now of 13 cases of varying severity, cases which I must consider sporadic cases, but one or two of which approached in severity what we see during epidemics exclusively, the foudroyant symptoms, the hemorrhages, the rapid collapse and sinking of the patient at the start of the disease. I mean the severity of the symptoms gradually increased so that, as in one case, it was five days before coma or sopor intervened.

The ages of the patients treated varied from three and one-half months to five and one-half and eleven years; three were below one year of age, and three were two years of age or younger. Of those below one year of age one was discharged cured at ten months of age. The others died. Of those from one year to two years of age, two of fifteen months, and one of two years, respectively, were cured; the remaining patients recovered.

In those children below one year of age who died, the youngest, three and one-half months of age, had been two weeks ill on admission, but was not by any means unconscious. The child received from 100 to 125 c.c. of serum. The temperature continued remittent, and was not in the least affected by the injections or punctures. The other case was admitted to the hospital twenty-two days after the onset of the disease, received four punctures and 66 c.c. of serum. The temperature could not be judged as being affected by the punctures in any way, as it was normal on admission. The child died a day or two after admission, and it is to be regretted that in both of these cases we did not get them at an earlier stage of the disease, as we cannot judge what would have been the effect had we received them at an early period. The first punctures in both cases were, of course, made immediately upon admission. The infant ten months of age, which recovered, was admitted fifteen days after the onset of the disease, with a temperature of 104°. A turbid fluid was obtained, and the child received 35 c.c. of serum. The temperature dropped from 104° to 98.8°, and the child was discharged cured clinically.

Of the other cases below two years of age and two years, the first punctures were made immediately after admission, and they had been ill from seven to twenty-three days. One was discharged as cured, but inasmuch as there was hydrocephalus present on discharge of the patient, I think it, being a posterior basic case, from a clinical standpoint cannot be said to have been completely cured. I would simply call it improved.

Of the patients above two years of age the time of illness on admission to the hospital varied from five days to fifteen days. They all received serum varying from 15 to 30 c.c. at each puncture, and some of them had as many as four punctures before the disease was considered under control. The fluid in most cases after the first puncture cleared up gradually, and in one case it is stated after the second puncture the cultures were sterile, and so with the third puncture, and in some cases after the fourth puncture. But it must be noted in spite of this fact the children were sick enough to be punctured not only on account of the run of the temperature, which was unchanged by the punctures, but the persistence of the hydrocephalus. This was especially marked in a boy of three years of age. The first puncture showed a white, cloudy fluid. Four punctures were made in this case, until the temperature would drop, and in all three punctures subsequent to the first the cultures and smears remained sterile. This should prove conclusively that the sterility of a fluid has very little to do with the clinical procedure in a given case, and I may say that in the epidemic a child mortally ill with meningitis would yield a fluid which was even cloudy, and the smears and cultures for some reason would remain sterile, and a subsequent puncture would show that there were meningococci present both in smear and culture, so that we have yet to learn a great deal as to why certain fluids are culturally sterile in a patient in whom a subsequent fluid will show meningococci, and also that the sterility of a fluid is not an indication that the patient necessarily does not need further puncture irrespective of serum.

The temperature after the injection of the serum in some of these cases fell by crisis from 104° to 98°. In one case it fell from 103° to 99° by lysis, and in one remaining case the puncture had no effect, and only fell and rose to a varying extent after the injections until either cured or fatal issue resulted. The amount of serum injected with punctures varied, and we can say in a general way that the amount of serum introduced equalled that of cerebrospinal fluid withdrawn from the patient. Some patients received one puncture, others as many as four, according to the necessities of the case.

The sickest child treated with the serum was a little girl four and one-half years of age. Hers was a case which approached in the picture, as nearly as we had seen in sporadic cases, the epidemic type of the disease. I saw her at her home. She was absolutely unconscious, paralytic on the right side of the body, and had a conjunctivitis as a result of her affection, with purulent discharge. She suffered from a double pneumonia, and had all the marked symptoms of cerebrospinal meningitis, with the exception of the hemorrhages. I gave, as my duty dictated, a grave prognosis, but advised immediate puncture. She was removed to the hospital, a great distance, and was immediately punctured and an injection of the serum introduced. In this case three punctures were made. It cannot be said that the temperature remained down for any length of time after any puncture, except after the second or third puncture. After the first puncture the temperature dropped from 104° to 98°; within thirty-six hours it rose again, and then after a second puncture it fell from 102° to 99° in twenty-four hours, and then rose again, and after the third puncture it fell gradually to 100°. This child gained consciousness after the first puncture; the hydrocephalus, however, persisted, and she was repeatedly punctured until she became rational after the third puncture. The second puncture was made two days after the first puncture; the third puncture was made four days after the second.

I have 13 patients thus far treated with the serum, two of which are under observation, two of which died; the remainder recovered with the exception of one, which was discharged improved.   A résumé of these cases will be given by Dr. Flexner in his complete report, and they are to be found under the heading of cases coming from the Mount Sinai Hospital.

I think it would be rather premature and unfair in every way to draw any conclusions as to the serum until we have seen a larger material and until we have tried it in an epidemic of the violent type, such as we passed through in 1904 and 1905.   On the other hand, it may be said that the serum of Flexner not only makes a very favorable impression, but is certainly a factor which cannot be excluded from the therapy of cerebrospinal meningitis, no matter what our subsequent conclusions may be.   It certainly does appear that with the serum as we perfect it we may have an improvement in the percentage of recoveries.   It is hard to say sincerely whether taking the cases I have treated I shall continue to have the same good fortune to save all but 2 cases of 13. Even if the cases I have lost were below one year of age, judging from the results obtained elsewhere, we may still meet with cases which we cannot save by the serum, and it would certainly be very unreasonable to expect a continuance of such a very high percentage of recoveries as we have just shown.

A CASE—APPARENTLY OF TUBERCULOUS MENINGITIS—IN WHICH THE AFTER HISTORY MAKES IT PROBABLE THAT THE DIAGNOSIS WAS MISTAKEN.

BY EDWARD M. BUCKINGHAM, M.D.,

Boston, Mass.

The patient, a boy of seventeen months, had malaise for one to two weeks, with cephalic cries. April 10th, Dr. J. W. Redmond was called because of some shuffling in walking, confined to one foot. No tenderness. In the next four days there were vomiting and convulsions. No history of tuberculosis nor of syphilis. Dr. Redmond asked me to see the child on the 14th. The difficulty in walking had then nearly disappeared; there was strabismus; the pupils were dilated and sluggish, the right being more dilated than the left. Knee jerks were unequal, the right being most marked. Kernig sign marked. Babinski present, but slight. Head not retracted. Ears and gums negative. Provisional diagnosis of tuberculous meningitis. Lumbar puncture was performed, the fluid running at first under considerable pressure; perhaps 10 or 12 c.c. withdrawn.

The pathological report by Dr. Leary is as follows: Specimen received from Dr. Redmond consists of 3½ c.c. of clear, colorless, watery fluid. This was shaken down in a centrifuge, without obtaining any visible sediment. The lower portions of fluid were smeared on slides and stained by Wright. Careful search resulted in the findings of eighty-nine cells, all but three of which were lymphoid cells. Diagnosis: Chronic inflammatory, probably tuberculous, meningitis.

The pressure symptoms were very quickly relieved, and in about a week the child had recovered health. He remained well May 20th, when Dr. Redmond last saw him. This after history is compatible with its being one of the comparatively few cases of cerebrospinal meningitis, in which there are prodromal symptoms and in which the cerebrospinal fluid contains an excess of mononuclear cells.

DISCUSSION OF PAPERS BY DRS. FLEXNER, CHURCHILL, DUNN, KNOX, HAND AND KOPLIK AT THE MEETING OF THE AMERICAN PEDIATRIC SOCIETY, MAY, 1908.

Dr. Holt.—Statistics were collected of 2,350 cases in the epidemic of 1904 in New York, of which the mortality, all non-serum treated, was 75 per cent. The most interesting part of the statistics was in the duration of the cases that recovered. Of 350 cases in which the duration of the disease was known, 50 per cent. lasted five weeks or longer. This is very striking in comparison with the cases reported to-day. During epidemic years we treated 83 and lost every case under one year of age, regardless of the type of the disease, frequency of lumbar puncture, or anything else. Unfortunately, there have been so few cases during the last year in New York that I have not seen many. I have seen 1 case of five months get well. It seems to me the showing here to-day is very encouraging.

Dr. Rotch.—I have had a very good opportunity for watching these cases, and would merely say I am very loath to speak of epidemic cases and sporadic cases; the special organism declares the disease. It may differ in type, but not in any essential way.

We have shown in our wards that these injections do no harm. In various successive years, trying all courses of treatment, antitoxins, vaccines and lumbar puncture, we have come to the conclusion that it is absolutely safe to give the injections, and, I think that is a very important point, because so much is said at times about it not being right to give them. We haven't time to wait; it is too serious a disease. We know what happens when we wait and when we do not take the cases early and give the injections. It seems to me absurd not to give the treatment at once, since we know that it does no harm.

In regard to the treatment with lumbar puncture, it certainly did at times do good temporarily—just as benefit would be had in relieving any pressure. Where there is an overwhelming number of organisms, drawing off a considerable amount of the fluid lessens the number of invaders, but that does not mean that there are not a large number still remaining which can get in their damaging work.

In the case of vaccines, we found that although not curative in any way, they did help in raising the opsonic index, but that is not of so much moment in the light of our recent views on the opsonic index. Something may be done with the vaccines, but not as much as with the serum.

Clinically, there is no doubt that we should repeat the dose. I believe that we may at times save life by injecting twice in the twenty-four hours. It seems to me that the consensus of this society should be to push the treatment. We may in this way, perhaps, arrest many of the sequelæ. We may be able to avoid these very distressing sequelæ which follow the fulminating cases. I am not afraid to give it and give it frequently. The youngest case I have seen was twenty-four hours old and died on the second day.

DR. JACOBI.—I have no active service and so I have no experience with the serum treatment of this disease. I know only what I have heard this morning and have read before.

One remark made this morning was that wherever there is a subnormal temperature there was a fatality. The question arises, can anything be done in those cases? Whenever we find a subnormal temperature in other septic diseases it is the result of a complication. It is so in diphtheria for instance. We expect an active case of diphtheria with subnormal temperature to die. These are the cases in which antitoxin is of no use no matter in what stage of the disease. In these cases there is a complication; a streptococcic infection for instance at the same time, and the question arises, Are not these cases with subnormal temperature due to a complication that we do not as yet understand, and could there not be a treatment besides the serum treatment in these cases to correct the complication? We know that a number of bad cases of diphtheria which are not benefited by antitoxin are still benefited by alcohol, which many of us have used for a number of years and a number of decades. A number of such cases will get well under attempted intoxication for these babies. The intoxication cannot be accomplished, but should be attempted. Give as large doses as will go down. Perhaps these cases of meningitis need to be treated with something else in conjunction with the serum; they may need to be stimulated.

I am delighted at what I have heard this morning, and sorry that I cannot contribute something more to the discussion along this line.

DR. MORSE.—My experience in the use of the serum has not been as great as that of some of the speakers, but I have seen a good deal of meningitis during the last ten years and have had some experience with the serum, especially in babies.

Knowing as we do how unreliable clinical observation is, it is conceivable that we may be mistaken in attributing the apparently good results to the serum, but we cannot be mistaken in what we see in the examination of the spinal fluid. When we see the organisms both within and without the cells and get a culture one day, and the next day, after giving the serum, find no organisms outside of the cells and a much smaller number in the cells and no growth on culture media, and the next day no organisms and negative cultures, we cannot doubt that the diminution and disappearance of the organisms are due to the serum.

It seems to me that the indication for lumbar puncture is the suspicion that the case may be meningitis. When there is any suspicion of meningitis it is our duty to do a puncture in order to find out. The indication for the use of serum is the presence of the meningococcus. If we get a turbid fluid we should, however, give the serum at once without waiting to determine whether or not the meningococcus is present, because if it is present much has been gained by giving the serum early, while if it is absent no harm is done.

It has been stated that the serum should not be given unless there are signs of increased cerebral pressure. It seems to me that this position is wrong and that it is the presence of the meningococcus, and not the presence or absence of increased cerebral pressure, which is the indication for the use of the serum. It has also been stated that we should put in the same amount of serum as of the fluid taken out. This does not seem rational, as, if there is increased pressure, the amount of fluid is abnormal and there is no reason for increasing the pressure again. The serum is given to kill the organisms and not to affect the pressure. In fact, in many cases the fontanel is depressed and yet the fluid is purulent and contains cocci. The serum should certainly be given in such cases. A dry tap, moreover, is not a contraindication for the giving of serum. I have recently had a case where a very thick fluid that would hardly run through the needle was obtained at the first puncture. This fluid showed the meningococcus, and the baby needed the serum. The punctures on the two following days were dry. The baby, nevertheless, needed the serum and got it. I agree heartily with Dr. Churchill that a turbid fluid is an indication for the use of the serum, and that the serum should be given early and often; certainly every day; sometimes oftener than once a day.

Dr. Freeman.—It seems to me that one point brought out today should be emphasized, and that is that the serum may be valuable in very late cases. In Dr. Churchill's cases there are two in which in a very late stage the serum was followed by prompt reaction.

Dr. W. W. Wilkinson (Guest), Washington.—In 10 cases treated in Washington at the Garfield Hospital. we had 7 recoveries and 3 deaths. Of the 3 cases that died, 1 had chronic hydrocephalus on admission and confirmed by autopsy. Of the other 2 cases, 1, I think, would possibly have recovered if larger amounts of the serum had been used in the beginning. 15 c.c. of serum were given at first; there was clinical improvement, and the serum was not repeated at that time. The organism reappeared in the fluid, however, and the patient died, despite repeated injections of the serum afterwards. Autopsy showed evidences of toxemia. The other case that died was a very severe one, and was in a comatose condition when the treatment was begun. There was considerable improvement in the meningeal symptoms and the spinal fluid following the administration of the serum, but he developed an intestinal paralysis and nothing could be done to save him.

In our cases we have had the best results with one injection of 15 c.c. or two of 30 c.c. on successive days. Four cases recovered with one injection only of 15 c.c. The earliest day we have gotten the cases has been the fourth. The duration of the cases following the injections has been about fourteen days, but in most of them there was a cessation of the bad symptoms in four or five days. In the studies we have made we invariably found the organisms rapidly disappearing from the fluid and the leukocytes diminished. We have also found an increase in phagocytosis; in some cases a very marked increase. The organism usually failed to grow and stained poorly, following the serum injections. One of the fatal cases was a mixed infection with the influenza bacillus.

Three cases recovered with sequelæ; 1 lost the right eye, 1 recovered with deafness and 1 with impaired mentality.

Dr. Adams.—I want to draw attention to the fact that while clinical observation may not be of much consequence, at the same time the results of clinical observation are of great importance. It has been shown here today that by the administration of this treatment we avoid those sequelæ, which are in many instances worse than death. In the observation of years we have learned that in institutions and in private practice a certain percentage die, and that of that percentage which is supposed to recover, many are not a complete recovery; they are deaf, blind or suffer from palsy or impaired mentality, and often it would have been better if they had died rather than to have been left as a burden on the community. From the results presented here today it would certainly seem that we may avoid a number of these misfortunes which have occurred under the other methods of treatment. Of course, with others, in following the previous methods of treatment, I have had a high mortality, corresponding to that given in the reports, and of those supposed to have recovered I have had a fair proportion of cases of deficient mentality and other sequelæ of the disease.

With the serum treatment my experience has been almost too limited to speak of, except that I had one child of seven months with pressure so great that it burst through the fontanel, and that child with one injection of the serum improved most markedly in twenty-four hours.

In another boy, thirteen years of age, the symptoms were

most intense, with convulsions and opisthotonos, and the boy recovered. The stiffness of the neck persisted for a couple of weeks, but he was perfectly conscious and intelligent.

Now there may be "doubting Thomases," but there has been proof enough here today to encourage us to go on with this treatment, which certainly offers much better results than any other method of treatment we have had in the past three decades.

Dr. Kerley.—I am sure you will all agree with me that this has probably been the most interesting session in the history of this Society. We have had brought before us here today a method for the treatment, alleviation and cure, largely the cure, of a disease that we have heretofore looked upon with little or no hope so far as medical means were concerned. I only hope that the good results that have been reported will be continued.

Dr. Knox.—I would like to add that in Baltimore the knowledge of the clinical value of the serum has attracted to the hospital for the spine very many more cases than we have formerly had. I think that should be generally emphasized. The health statistics in Baltimore show that there have been no more cases than usual; no epidemic.

Dr. Dunn.—I just want to say one or two words in explanation. I was interested in hearing Dr. Knox say the serum gave a good deal of pain. I saw that in 2 cases; the patients complained of severe pain in the back of the legs and knees, but most of them did not make this complaint. I found that in these 2 cases I had failed to warm the serum. I do not know whether that had anything to do with it or not, but the majority of my cases did not complain of pain.

In regard to Dr. Jacobi's remarks I did not mean to say that all cases with subnormal temperature died; in fact, 1 case recovered after seven weeks' illness who had subnormal temperature. I meant that all cases that had passed over the period of active fever and symptoms frequently go into a state of unconsciousness with subnormal temperature, and that that was the type of case that was unfavorable.

I would say, too, that so far as our cases in the last ten years are concerned, we have not been able to observe any difference in type in the so-called epidemic years.

Dr. Koplik.—I would say only one word more. I still believe that we should never puncture except on indication, and that we do not want *only* to diminish pressure by puncture, but we wish also to affect the meningococci. In these cases I have observed that if you introduce 30 c.c. after having withdrawn that amount, the next day, the indication of the amount of fluid in the ventricle is less than the preceding day. For that reason, the child doing well, I think it superfluous therapy to puncture daily unless the symptoms warrant it.

Dr. Simon Flexner, New York (closing discussion).—I recognize the criticism Dr. Koplik makes, that meningitis is a very variable disease; it may not only vary in different seasons, but in different localities. It has not been possible in every instance to get comparative statistics; that is, cases occurring at the same time and of the same age, where nothing, or only lumbar puncture has been done and then those in which the serum has been used systematically.

The largest and the best statistics I have gotten from Belfast, and this is fortunate, because it has been for a year past passing through an epidemic. During the height of the epidemic a mortality of 75 per cent. was reported. I cannot say whether lumbar puncture was used only for diagnostic purposes or also as a therapeutic measure. Dr. Robb has secured for me a record of cases treated outside of the fever hospitals during the same period as those treated with serum in the hospitals. The mortality had been 80 per cent. at a time when it was only 26 per cent. in the hospitals. Of course, the cases outside were probably not treated so well as those in the hospitals. There is also this difference to consider, that the cases outside may have included a greater number of fulminating examples, but the difference between 80 per cent. and 26 per cent. is so great that something else than this must be invoked to explain it. Akron, O., passed through a small epidemic the year after the New York one. There were 26 cases there and in the surrounding locality considerably more. Two sets of figures are to be considered here—12 cases treated with the serum with 3 deaths and 9 recoveries, and 9 cases treated without the serum with 8 deaths and 1 recovery.

I only state these points for what they are worth. I do not wish to be put in the position of making out an overstrong case for the serum, though I believe in it.

As to the manner of production of the serum, the serum belongs to the class of bacteriolytic sera, in which we are obliged to use the entire constituents of the organisms in its preparation. We know now at least three antitoxic bacterial sera—of diphtheria, tetanus and dysentery. They are the most useful; we all know what they accomplish. You can give an animal any amount of tetanus toxin you please, and if you give a corresponding amount of antitoxin the animal will be saved. The same thing appears to be true of the dysenteric serum. If you multiply the toxic and antitoxic sera equally you secure neutralization. This is not true of the antimeningitis serum. In making the serum the organisms are subjected to unfavorable conditions, when they undergo autolysis and yield an extracellular toxin. With that preparation the process of immunization of horses is begun. It takes many months to accustom the horses to a considerable dose. After this the living organisms are employed to secure the full value of the microorganisms' immunization.

Now when you test the serum on animals, it is found that it does not produce neutralization of the toxin according to the law of multiples, as is the case in the diphtheric and tetanic sera. The guinea pig can be protected up to a certain amount, but a point is quickly reached beyond which multiples of the serum do not neutralize.

In employing a serum of this class it should be borne in mind that the results depend, to a considerable degree, on the concentration. The antibody should be present in a certain state of concentration. When it is diluted too much by the blood and lymph it is powerless to produce the most favorable results.

I believe that the success which has been achieved by this serum has been in virtue of the fact that you bring a bacteriolytic and somewhat antitoxic substance in contact with the focus of the disease. I think this the secret of the matter so far as efficiency goes. Given into the circulation the secretion into the subdural space is slow and imperfect. The thing to be emphasized is that you require this fluid in a certain high state of concentration, and hence injections made directly into the spinal membranes is the obvious way of accomplishing this desideratum.

There is a larger question involved in this study, which is that it is an indication of the value of local application of antisera. If a means could be found of treating pneumonia by some such method as this it would be one of the things by all means to be tried. To return to meningitis. In employing the antiserum, your problem is not to neutralize a poison that is already attached to the viscera. The poison of the diplococcus is not a general, systemic one, but a local one, chiefly acting on the nervous system. Hence the endeavor to bring the agent directly in contact with the focus of the disease, which idea involves, I believe, a slight departure from the general notion of the manner in which infectious processes are influenced by curative sera. The reason we have failed with sera in certain diseases is perhaps because we have tried to reach the local processes through the general circulation. Now in meningitis the general viscera show few evidences of injury at autopsy, thus supporting the notion that the systemic effects of the poison are inconspicuous.

A REPORT UPON ONE THOUSAND TUBERCULIN TESTS IN YOUNG CHILDREN.

BY L. EMMETT HOLT, M.D., LL.D.,

Professor of Diseases of Children in the College of Physicians and Surgeons,
Columbia University, New York.

The observations included in the following report were all made at the Babies' Hospital upon ward patients. Very few of the children were over three years of age, the majority being under two years. Nearly all of the observations have been made in the past year. I desire at the outset to express my indebtedness to Dr. Josephine Hemenway, house physician at the Babies' Hospital, for her invaluable assistance in the work, the results of which are embodied in this paper. In the early part of the year, unless some positive contraindication existed, some test, most frequently the eye test, was used as a routine measure, in order to determine whether and under what circumstances reactions were obtained in healthy children or in those at least presumably non-tubercular. During the latter half of the period the tests have been chiefly used when some grounds for suspecting tuberculosis existed. Routine tests proved of considerable value in revealing cases of tuberculosis not hitherto suspected. A positive reaction to a skin or eye test was immediately followed up by careful clinical study of the case to discover, if possible, any other evidence of tuberculosis. In a large proportion of such patients bacilli were found in the sputum; though in many only after prolonged search and repeated examinations, thus establishing the accuracy and the value of the test. In many patients further evidence was afforded by the development of definite signs of pulmonary disease.

The Ophthalmic Reaction.—The ophthalmic test was made 615 times; in most instances one test only was made in a patient, although in a few children, where the results were questionable, the test was repeated. The ophthalmic tests were all made with tuberculin obtained from the Rockefeller Institute, which had been precipitated with 65 per cent. alcohol. Before using it was freshly

dissolved in a sterile saline solution. For the first half of these
tests a 1 per cent. solution was used, for the latter half a ½
per cent. Especial care was taken not to use the tuberculin in
an eye which was the seat of any form of disease, tuberculous
or otherwise. As a further precaution the hands of the children
were confined during the first twelve hours to prevent any rub-
bing of the eye.

RESULTS IN 615 OPHTHALMIC TESTS.

Pathological Condition.		Positive Reactions.	Negative Reactions.	Doubtful Reactions.
Positive tuberculosis	38	25	10	3
(Autopsy or bacilli in sputum.)			(9 dying or extremely sick children.)	
Probable tuberculosis	21	19	..	?
(Evidence: Other tuberculin reactions, history or physical signs)				
Probably *not* tuberculosis..	555		546	7
				(All slight.)
Positively not tuberculosis..	1		..	
(Autopsy.)				
Totals.......	615	47	556	12

In the preceding table are given the reactions in the different
types of cases. In the group marked *probably not tuberculosis*
are included those in which no evidence of tuberculosis existed
other than the reaction.

The clinical course which the reaction follows is its most
diagnostic feature and hence rather close observation of a patient
is necessary or some of the milder reactions will be missed. There
is usually congestion of the conjunctiva, with some swelling and
an increased secretion of mucus, which is frequently very
abundant, so that the lids are adherent. There are very seldom
pus cells and repeated cultures made revealed no micro-organ-
isms. The symptoms usually begin in from six to eight hours
after the tuberculin is used and reach their height in the first
twenty-four hours, gradually fading. The usual duration of
symptoms is from one to three days. In about 12 per cent. of
the cases the reaction lasted somewhat longer than three days; in
one case it lasted ten days, but in no case was the test followed
by any unpleasant results. Having the opposite eye for comparison enables one, in most cases, to be certain as to the existence

of a reaction. There were, however, a few cases in which the symptoms were so slight that the results must be classed as doubtful.

I am aware that serious results with the ophthalmic test have occasionally been reported by other observers. The precautionary measures taken in this group of cases are, I believe, of considerable importance and largely responsible for our freedom from unpleasant results. On account of the kind of observation necessary, and the possible dangers connected with the eye test, it is not wise to employ it indiscriminately as among the outpatients of a hospital.

The statement has been repeatedly made that young infants do not respond to the eye test. Such was not our experience. Of this series of cases positive reactions were obtained in 14 patients under one year old, 6 of whom were under six months and 1 only two months old. So far as we could see, the character of the reaction and the frequency with which it occurred were not affected by the age of the patients nor by the extent nor activity of the pathological process, but only by the susceptibility of the patient. In no cases were positive reactions obtained in dying children or those suffering from extreme prostration. In this respect it corresponded with the other tests.

The Skin Reaction.—The skin test of Von Pirquet was employed 217 times. It was made with crude tuberculin obtained from the laboratory of the New York Health Department, which was simply diluted with sterile water to a 25 per cent. strength. With a sterile needle three short linear scratches were made, usually upon the extensor surface of the forearm and into the middle one the tuberculin was rubbed. The skin was allowed to dry and in some cases was covered for a few hours with a piece of sterile gauze. The first sign of reaction was usually apparent in from six to twelve hours; rarely later than twenty-four hours. There is seen a rather bright aureola slowly spreading from the line of scarification to a distance, varying with the intensity of the reaction, from $1/16$ to $1/4$ inch. The more pronounced reactions are accompanied by an induration readily palpable. The reaction reaches its height in most cases in from twenty-four to thirty-six hours. It then fades rather slowly, usually lasting two or three days, but not infrequently for a week or even longer. It may be followed by a slight desquamation.

Vesiculation was not observed. Although it varied considerably in intensity the reaction was generally perfectly definite and in no instance was the result considered doubtful.

In the following table is given a summary of the reactions obtained in the different pathological conditions. As in the table of ophthalmic reactions, *probably not tuberculosis* signifies no other evidence of tuberculosis than the reaction to the test:—

RESULTS IN 217 SKIN TESTS (VON PIRQUET).

Pathological Condition.	Positive Reactions.	Negative Reactions.
Positive tuberculosis ..... 22 (Sputum, autopsy or operation.)	12	10 (9 dying or extremely sick children; 1 cured.
Probable tuberculosis ..... 20 (Evidence: Other tests, history or physical signs.)	15	5
Probably not tuberculosis..172	6	166
Positively not tuberculosis.. 3 (Autopsy.)	..	3
Totals....... 217	33	184

The reaction in general corresponded with the pathological condition, the exceptions being in the second and third groups of cases in which we had no means of determining definitely as to the reliability of the reaction.

The skin test possesses the great advantage of ease of application, of not requiring close observation, and of freedom from unpleasant or serious consequences. In no instance was any trouble seen from the inoculation or any excessive reaction. With the two scarifications for control there seemed little difficulty in recognizing a positive reaction; whereas, in the eye there were a certain number of cases in which doubt existed as to whether or not enough disturbance was seen to be called a reaction.

The Puncture Reaction.—When tuberculin is injected to secure the fever reaction in doses ranging from $1/_{10}$ mgr. to 5 mgr., no local reaction is observed if the injections are made deeply into the muscles. If, however, they are made subcutaneously a local reaction is regularly seen in cases in which a positive fever reaction occurs. This phenomenon, first observed by Epstein, afterward by Schick, is known as the "stich-reaction." In 38 cases tuberculin was injected subcutaneously for the purpose of obtaining this puncture reaction. The usual dose employed for this purpose was $^1/_{100}$ mgr. These patients were all submitted previously or subsequently to Von Pirquet's skin test. The skin reaction corresponded in every instance with the puncture reaction, hence it seems unnecessary to tabulate the cases separately. With the dose mentioned, the puncture reaction was not so marked as when a larger dose (½ mgr. or 1 mgr.) was used. The conclusion drawn from this limited experience was that the puncture test possessed no advantages over the scarification test and that it was somewhat more troublesome of application.

Fever Reaction to Tuberculin Injections.—This is quite as reliable in young children as in older patients. The fever test is limited in its application since most cases of active tuberculosis at this period of life are accompanied by fever. Furthermore, young children have slight rises of temperature from so many causes that unless the reaction is decided and typical in its course the result may be doubtful. I have not considered a reaction definite unless the temperature has reached at least 102°F. It is necessary that the temperature be taken at four-hour intervals before the injection is given and after the injection at two-hour intervals. Accurate dosage is a matter of much importance. Very small doses are unreliable and too large doses may be fraught with some risk. After considerable experimenting I have settled upon the doses of ½ mgr. for infants under six months and 1 mgr. for those who are older.

Injections of tuberculin in patients suspected to be tuberculous were employed 130 times. For the most part, the injections were made deeply into the muscles and no local reactions were observed. The temperature usually began to rise in from six to twelve hours, reaching its maximum in from four to eight hours. The average maximum reaction was 103.3°, which was reached on the average in thirteen hours. The temperature remained near the highest point for from six to eight hours and then rather rapidly fell to the normal. As a rule, the larger the dose given the more rapid the reaction and the higher the temperature. In no case were any serious symptoms observed to follow the injection, although in several instances high temperatures were accompanied by discomfort, restlessness and other symptoms indicating a constitutional disturbance of some severity. In no instance was it apparent that the injection had resulted in the lighting up of a latent tuberculous process. In a few instances a general erythema was noticed as after diphtheria antitoxin.

The results of the injections in the various pathological conditions are shown in the following table:—

RESULTS OF 130 TUBERCULIN INJECTIONS.

Pathological Condition.		Positive Reactions.	Negative Reactions.	Doubtful Reactions.
Positive tuberculosis 28		22	2	4
(Sputum, autopsy, operation or c. s. fluid.)			(In 1 patient apparently cured.)	
Probable tuberculosis 21		18	3	
(Evidence: Other tests, history or physical signs.)				
Probably *not* tuberculosis.. 80			78	
Positively *not* tuberculosis.. 1		1	..	..
(Autopsy.)				
Totals....... 130		42	83	5

On the whole the results obtained by the different tests corresponded with each other and with the pathological condition as determined by other means, the only notable exception being that dying children or those who were extremely sick did not, as a rule, react to any of the tests. An attempt has been made to compare the reliability of the different tests by grouping the exceptional reactions observed in 16 cases in the following table. The numbers, however, are too small to admit of any very definite conclusions.

It will be seen that some failures and some unexplained reactions occurred with all of the tests. The results with any test cannot therefore be regarded as conclusive, although a positive reaction creates a very strong probability that tuberculosis is present. This is increased if the result is confirmed by other tests.

In reliability there is not much to choose between the skin and eye tests. The skin reaction is, I think, more characteristic and less likely to be doubtful than are some of the eye reactions. Some instances of doubt must occur in the temperature reactions on account of the liability of small children to slight rises of temperature from minor digestive disturbances or other causes.

In ease of application there is a decided advantage in the skin test. The scarification is a trifling thing. The patient does not require continuous observation before or after, and the reaction lasts for a considerable time. The ophthalmic cases need closer watching, the reaction is shorter and may be missed. It cannot well be used in ambulatory patients. The puncture test is slightly more of an operation and may be objected to. The fever reaction is only admissible when the child can be under very close observation.

Objectionable features are wanting in the skin test. There is no local discomfort, no general reaction, and I have seen no complications. With proper precautions I believe the eye test to be quite safe, although an intense or prolonged reaction sometimes occurs which is not pleasant to see; besides, in pathological conditions of the eye disastrous results may follow. However the eye is too delicate and important an organ to be used for a test when any other will answer quite as well. For general use the skin test is to be advised in preference.

With the temperature reaction we may get accompanying the fever constitutional symptoms which are quite disagreeable. There exists a possibility that a latent process may be lighted up. With mistakes in dosage which have been made, serious consequences may follow. These risks are added objections to the use of this test. It is certainly an advantage to have several tests both for purposes of confirmation and to use one where another is not applicable. For all tests one must be sure as to the purity, strength and freshness of the tuberculin used.

All of these tests have been too recently introduced for the final word to be spoken regarding them. No one of them is absolutely conclusive as is the demonstration of the tubercle bacillus in the sputum, cerebro-spinal fluid or elsewhere, and one should not fall into the error of depending upon the local tests to the neglect of other means of diagnosis, even though the search for the tubercle bacillus involves greater labor. In general, while the tests furnish strong probability of the existence of a tuberculous lesion, they do not enable us to distinguish between a latent and an active condition. This may at times be confusing. A child may give a positive skin or eye reaction when suffering from an

EXCEPTIONAL REACTIONS IN 16 CASES.

(− =negative reaction; + =positive; ?=doubtful.)

I. POSITIVE TUBERCULOSIS WITH NEGATIVE OR CONTRADICTORY REACTIONS.

	Age	History and Clinical Diagnosis	Eye	Skin	Puncture	Fever	
1	20 mos.	Bronchopneumonia; bacilli in sputum.	− to 1% − to 1%	−			First eye test in January skin and second eye test in May, shortly befor death.
2	6 mos.	Chronic costosternal abscess; bacilli in discharge.				− to 1/10 mgr. (twice) − to 1 mgr. + to 1 " (102° in 13 hrs.) ? 3 mgr. (103° in 24 hrs.)	Had croup at time las test was made. Died o diphtheria 5 month later. Abscess ne healed.
3	4 years	Tuberculous glands; operation.	− to ½%	+			Skin test 1 month la than eye.

	Age	History and Clinical Diagnosis	Eye	Skin	Puncture	Fever	Remarks
4	3 years	Bronchopneumonia; empyema; recovery; father tuberculous.	− to ½% − to 1%	+	+		Apparently well 5 month after attack.
5	3 years	Unresolved broncho-pneumonia.	+ to 1%	+	+	− to 1 mgr.	Three months later chil apparently well.
6	14 mos.	Bronchitis; large abdomen; tubercular peritonitis. (?)			+	− to 1/10 mgr. + to 1 mgr. (104.4° in 13 hrs.)	Following second injec tion a local reaction oc curred at site of first on made 10 days before Lost sight of.
7	4 years	Chronic Bronchitis; signs cleared up.	+ to ½% Feb.	+ Feb. (twice) − July	+ June	+ Feb. (three times) + June	Following tuberculin in jection in June, typica reaction in eye in whi tuberculin was used months before.
8	4 years	Anemia, malnutrition; no pulmonary signs. (Sister died of tubercular meningitis.)		+		− to 1 mgr.	Lost sight of.

acute pulmonary disease which by its course is shown to be non-tuberculous, although grave suspicion of acute pulmonary tuberculosis may have existed and apparently be confirmed by the tuberculin tests. Much needless alarm may therefore be produced by a positive reaction, which really indicates only that somewhere the child has a tuberculous focus but does not prove that his present disease is of a tuberculous nature. While of the greatest assistance in diagnosis, the various tests are always to be taken in connection with the general symptoms and the physical signs. Taken apart from them, however, they may be very misleading.

14 West 55th St., New York.

III. PROBABLY NOT, OR WITH NO OTHER EVIDENCE OF, TUBERCULOSIS, BUT WITH POSITIVE OR CONTRADICTORY REACTIONS.

ase	Age	History and Clinical Diagnosis	Eye	Skin	Puncture	Fever	Remarks
9	10 mos.	Pyemic abscesses.	+ to ½% – to 1%	–			Fat, well nourished chil
10	9 mos.	Bronchitis; recovery; well nourished child.	+ to ½% (April)	– April – July		+ ¼ mgr. (102.4° in 14 hrs.)	Child well 3 months aft test.
11	9 mos.	Unresolved bronchopneumonia.	– to ½%	– (twice)		+ ¼ mgr. (104° in 8 hrs)	Lost sight of.
12	22 mos.	Bronchopneumonia; sequel of measles; general condition bad; sputum neg.	+ to ½%	–	– (twice)		Died. No autopsy.
13	3 years	Chronic bronchitis; no family history.		+	+	– to 1 mgr.	Poorly nourished child, but running about. Reported well 5 mos. later.
14		Malnutrition and gastroenteritis; family history negative.		+ (twice)		– to 1 mgr.	No pulmonary signs 2 weeks later. Lost sight of.

	Age	History and Clinical Diagnosis	Eye	Skin	Puncture	Fever	Remarks
15	7 mos.	Bronchopneumonia; autopsy.	+ to ½%				Many sputum examinations all negative. In good condition at time of test.
16	17 mos.	Bronchopneumonia; autopsy.				– to 1/10 mgr. – to 1 mgr. + to 5 mgr. (102° in 21 hrs.)	Condition good at first two tests; bad at last test.

DISCUSSION.

DR. NORTHRUP.—My conclusions have been the same as those of Dr. Holt.

In regard to the injection test some years ago, under the direction of Dr. Trudeau, I carried out at the Presbyterian Hospital 65 tests on adults, and I should not take such a cheerful view of this test as does Dr. Holt, because it made these people so very sick. I consider that there was some risk in the test as administered at that time.

With regard to the eye test, when Dr. Holt has had his first accident he will take a little less positive view about that test. I have not personally had such, but have seen an unfavorable reaction in a public institution, in which there was proper dosage, administered in a proper way, but the child reacted in a very bad way.

With regard to the skin test, in a talk with Dr. Baldwin, of Saranac, in the early part of this month, he suggested that there should be three little points of scarification, and for that we adopted a modification of the instrument used by Dr. Trudeau—a

screw· driver such as our wives use for their eye-glasses. It removes just enough of the superficial skin to make a uniform little
round place, making three of them. Dr. Baldwin suggested using
a broth for the first; broth plus the old tuberculin, 5 per cent. for
the second; and, plus tuberculin 10 per cent. for the third. This
method of administration will furnish control and two degrees
of reaction in the skin.

DR. ROTCH.—We have been carrying on the various tuberculin tests quite extensively in Boston and have certain men
especially connected with carrying out these tests. One of
them is one of my assistants in the Children's Hospital. A great
deal has been done at the Massachusetts Hospital, and I have
had Dr. Floyd take charge of the tests among the children.
We have a great deal of material. There has been established
a special dispensary for tuberculosis, which is in charge of some
of our best men and on one of the days the material is derived
entirely from children. I have control of that day and have
placed Dr. Floyd and Dr. Bowditch in charge. These cases are
of special interest because they are a class in which the tuberculin
test is required to make the diagnosis. They are what we call
closed cases of tuberculosis; where careful study has led us to
believe that they are tuberculous, but where the diagnosis is very
difficult to establish with the usual methods of examination. For
instance, in the light forms of miliary tuberculosis, with nothing
very marked and where there is no sputum. or where the disease
has not progressed far enough to enable us in any other way than
with the Roentgen ray to distinguish the disease. This material
we have under close observation. Having been fairly diag-
nosticated the children are then forwarded to my wards in the
Children's Hospital, where they are kept a few days, the diagnosis
carefully gone over and substantiated and then they are sent out
to another hospital of which I have complete control, with sixty
or eighty beds, and where I have 20 of these cases of closed
tuberculosis under my eye all the time. Dr. Floyd has charge and
administers the treatment. That is the material from which I
draw my conclusions.

The temperature test will probably not be so popular, as Dr.
Holt has said, in the future as the eye or skin tests, because there
are a large number of cases in which we are doubtful whether we
are dealing with tuberculosis or not, in which we want to make
the test and are unable to do so because the temperature interferes
with the test. Whatever the disease, tubercular or non-tubercular, the temperature test cannot be used in a very large number
of cases. We have to wait until the temperature is fairly normal
—99° or 100°—otherwise the test is interfered with. We are still
a little uncertain as to whether the temperature test, when it can
be used, does not give us more exact results than the others. That
has not been proven with us yet, and I am glad to know what Dr.
Holt has done in this respect. In regard to whether there is any

danger in the temperature test, we have never met with any serious results, except where there has been a fault in the technique. The children do, as Dr. Northrup has said, have more or less ill effects from the injection test, but not in any way to compare with what he has suggested. If the adult patients suffer so much it is different with the children. We have never hesitated to give the test where we can. The child will perhaps have a little malaise and a certain amount of erythema at times.

When we come to the eye test, we have never seen any bad results. I have had one of my assistants, Dr. Lucas, give it in 100 consecutive cases without reference to tuberculosis, and it seldom gave a reaction where there was not tuberculosis, and in almost every case disclosed the tuberculosis.

In regard to the skin test, we are having a great deal of it done, and we hope that will be the test we can use, because it makes a great deal of difference as to the rapidity with which we can make the test and get results.

As to injections, Dr. Floyd, and those who are carrying out these investigations, give the small doses, frequently repeated, in their tests.

DR. CAILLÉ.—This is a very important and practical communication and I desire to put myself on record as opposed to the eye test. My first introduction to an eye test was six years ago while a guest of Prof. Dunbar in Hamburg, when he was investigating hay-fever, he being a sufferer himself. He placed some pollen poison into his eye and some into mine. His eye became red almost at once; he applied the antibody and the eye cleared up. The pollen poison did not affect my eye. I told him then that I did not think the eye was a proper organ for experimentation and he partly agreed with me.

The tuberculin test we have used in about 60 cases and have found it a failure in about 5 per cent. of cases. It has a peculiar way of acting; for instance, in 2 cases of tuberculous peritonitis that came to operation on the same day and were proven to be tuberculous by direct inspection, one showed the reaction and the other did not. A case of miliary tuberculosis did not react. In fact, the advanced cases failed to react. An advanced case of ankle tuberculosis did not react while a mild case did react after a second injection. We think it fairly unreliable and in a general way I am opposed to the eye test.

DR. HENRY KOPLIK.—We have been using the injection test several years. We have found the Von Pirquet test useful in those cases where fever exists and the tuberculin injection is ruled out. The primary dose we use is much smaller than that recommended by Dr. Holt and smaller than we are accustomed to seeing described in articles on the subject. We use $^1/_{10}$ mg. and run it up as indicated. We have been applying the Von Pirquet test during the past year and have quite a number of cases that will be published at the Tuberculosis Congress. We find it quite reliable and convenient in those cases where the injections are not applicable. We have had no ill results. We use one positive scarification and two controls—one with salt solution and one with carbolized glycerin.

The eye test I have not allowed in my service from the start. In New York we have had 2 cases in adults in which the eyes were practically ruined by the test. They were in cases not suited for the test; one had a chorioditis and the other tubercular nodules. Both patients lost their eyes. I never allow it to be used because I am afraid of it. You cannot always tell in a baby whether the eye is sound or not and I take no chances.

I would report the following case: I was asked by a physician to see a baby which showed no clinical signs of tuberculosis. It had gone through a slight grippe attack and was running a little temperature. The eye test was applied by another in this child and a most violent reaction resulted and the child was labeled as acutely tuberculous and you can imagine the panic in that family. I could not find any signs of tuberculosis from a clinical standpoint and there was slight leukocytosis, which would be against a diagnosis of tuberculosis. The child finally recovered a week or two after, gained five pounds and regained a normal color and was apparently well. Such a child might later show that the test was correct, but that has nothing to do with the embarrassing position in which the physician and family were placed, and I would be very opposed to taking an exceptional chance of being placed in such a position.

DR. HAMILL.—In the course of the last winter I have applied the conjunctival test of Calmette and Wolff-Eisner; the scarification test of Von Pirquet and the Moro ointment test to a large number of cases. It was my desire to determine the relative value of the various tests, because I had the feeling that the eye test produced a baneful and disturbing lesion and, owing to the delicate structure of the eye, it might not be free of danger. My preconceived idea of the eye test, I regret to state, was confirmed in my results.

In the 177 cases in which I used it, there were 8 severe complications. It is only just to state that I was working with institutional children, whilst, on the other hand, every effort was made to carefully select the cases and none was used in which there was any known contraindication. When complications occurred, they were promptly placed under the care of Dr. Shumway, the ophthalmologist of the institution.

Of the 8 complications, there were 2 showing severe persistent purulent conjunctivitis, 5 phlyctenules and 1 an iridocyclitis with a central corneal ulcer of such size that there will result a scar which must permanently interfere with vision. I desire, therefore, to protest against the employment of this test.

Unquestionably, Dr. Holt has been applying the test to a better class of children than those with whom I worked, but, when it is considered that in my 177 cases I obtained positive results in 70 per cent., it is very evident that the chances of complication were greater and that the results are not, therefore, entirely comparable.

In 144 of the 177 cases in which the eye test was applied, I also employed the scarification and ointment tests. In the earlier cases I applied first the eye test, next the scarification test and finally the ointment test. In the majority of cases the latter two were applied at the same time, and in the last groups examined, the three tests were applied at the same time.

The most interesting feature of my results and that which I started out to determine was the uniformity of reaction, as well as uniformity in the degree of reaction. In 35 per cent. of the cases reaction was most marked with the scarification test; in 34 per cent. most marked with the conjunctival test, and in 24 per cent. with the ointment test. In 85 of the 177 cases the subcutaneous test was applied in order to confirm the results. This was accomplished in all but one case. In the earlier cases I gave but $^1/_{10}$ mg. subcutaneously; failing to obtain a reaction in a number of cases, I increased the dose to $\frac{1}{2}$ mg., using as much as $\frac{3}{4}$ mg. in the last group tested.

The striking uniformity of reaction makes it evident that the eye test has no advantages over the others and further emphasizes the importance of eliminating this method of applying tuberculin. I deferred the physical examination of the children on whom I used these tests until the results of the tests had been determined for two reasons—first, in order to avoid being prejudiced in my interpretation of the reactions, and, second, to make me especially careful in making the physical examinations of those cases which reacted. The results of the physical examination of the cases showed 13 cases of tuberculosis; 23 with signs suspicious of tuberculosis; the remainder being clinically non-tuberculous.

Of the 23 suspicious cases all but one reacted positively; of the 13 who were definitely tuberculous, all reacted positively. Of the total number of cases, as has been previously said, 70 per cent. showed positive reactions. The cause of this high percentage is attributable to the fact that I was working with children living in a very much overcrowded, very badly ventilated institution, in which there were a number of cases of well-defined tuberculosis scattered throughout the various dormitories and in which there are probably some tuberculous cases amongst the attendants.

I observed one well-defined late reaction following the Moro ointment test, which persisted at its maximum for about three weeks. Following the suggestion of Daels, who studied the late reactions following the scarification test, I had sections cut from papules taken from these delayed reactions, as well as some papules taken from a case giving a prompt reaction. These sections showed simple infiltration of the skin, whilst those of Daels reproduced the histology of the tubercle which he proved to be due to the presence of particles of dead bacilli in the tuberculin which he used.   The tuberculin with which I worked had been thrice filtered through a Berkefelde filter of the fine flow and could, therefore, not have contained any of the particles of tubercles.

In one group of 24 cases, I applied both the human and bovine tuberculin by the scarification method.   In 3 instances there was no reaction to either.   In 9 reaction was more marked to the human; in 2 instances it was positive to the human and negative to the bovine; in 8 the reaction was the same in both, and in 2 instances it was more marked to the bovine.   This latter point may be of no special significance, except that the bovine tuberculin is relatively weaker than the human, because the tuberculins are not prepared from weighed amounts.   The cultures which are used are taken from the surface of the bouillon.   The human culture grows much more luxuriantly than the bovine, in consequence of which the quantity of bacilli obtained is greater and will, therefore, produce a larger amount of tuberculin.   Aside from this, in comparing these tests, I applied the human tuberculin to 2 points, whilst the bovine was applied to but one.   I did this with the idea of acting to the disadvantage of the bovine tuberculin.

DR. WENTWORTH.—I would call attention to the positive reactions in the healthy cases.   There are a good many tables published in the German literature of healthy persons giving a positive reaction.   In one series one-sixth of the cases gave a positive reaction for the eye test and almost one-half for the cutaneous test.   How they proved them to be non-tuberculous I am not sure.

Wolff-Eisner claims priority over Calmette for the eye test by several weeks.   He referred to the matter in a discussion some weeks before Calmette published his article.

DR. L. EMMETT HOLT (closing discussion).—Dr. Park tells me that no deductions are to be drawn between the results of one man using ½ per cent. and another using 1 per cent. tuberculin, because it differs so in strength.

Regarding Dr. Wentworth's point as to a positive reaction in healthy persons, I wonder if he has seen the recent article in which statistics are given comparing the tests with an equal number of autopsies, the point being to determine the latent tuberculosis.   In these cases the latent tuberculosis steadily rises from the first few months to past fourteen, and in the autopsy cases the frequency rises at fourteen years.   We were very careful in our tests if we got a positive reaction to find out if the patient had tuberculosis or not.   I would emphasize the importance of studying the sputum, going over the case again and again until certain.

Dr. Koplik raised an interesting point in connection with the possibility of getting the reaction in a non-tuberculous patient. That doesn't simply apply to the eye tests, but to all the tests. We are confronted with a difficult situation. We apply the tests and get a positive reaction; the child's symptoms clear up and he is apparently well; but that proves nothing, except that the disease he was having at the time was not due to a tuberculous lesion. I think it is important for the people to know so that they may be warned in time of the existence of a latent tuberculosis in order that they may take proper steps toward its treatment. We should apply the test in doubtful cases, but should be careful to discriminate between a latent tuberculosis and another existing infection.

A SIMPLE METHOD OF CIRCUMCISION IN THE NEWBORN.

BY W. REYNOLDS WILSON, M.D.,

Philadelphia.

In carrying out the operation of circumcision in the newly born, simplicity in operation should be kept in view. By comparing the usual method with that about to be described it will be seen that the latter is to be recommended because it conforms to this requirement. Pursuing this comparison further we may note the disadvantages of the usual method, supposing this to be by clamping the prepuce and cutting away the redundant portion with a knife, the skin and mucous membrane afterward being secured by sutures. The first of these disadvantages lies in the incompleteness of the removal of the foreskin in instances where the latter is adherent to the glans. When the clamp is applied the prepuce becomes drawn forward in a roll; the knife may thus remove only a circular band of skin while that portion of the foreskin contiguous with the opening remains. This will, therefore, have to be trimmed away after removal of the clamp. It is, however, in the application of the sutures that the greatest disadvantage lies. The primary object of these is to secure the attachment of the skin to the mucous membrane. Incidentally the control of bleeding is accomplished by the pressure of the sutures. Unfortunately this is not always the case, and it may require a number of sutures to control the bleeding points. The sutures are thus placed irregularly and may have to be tightened to the point of unduly constricting the tissues. As a result edema occurs and the sutures begin to cut. The indentation of the coronal edge of the prepuce which follows and the persistent edema make the results of the operation unsightly. Should any of the sutures become infected a slough may form and the resulting granulation may be more or less difficult to deal with, owing to the adhesion of the dressing to the surface of the wound. The length of time also required for a painstaking suturing of the skin and mucous membrane prolongs the operation unduly, considering it as a simple operation.

In contrast to this the method about to be described presents many advantages. No claim for originality can be put forward in respect to this procedure, as it follows in technic that used in the Hebrew rite with a certain exception. According to the Hebrew method the foreskin is removed by a single sweep of the knife. This requires skill, and when properly done removes exactly that portion of the prepuce which has interfered with retraction. The writer has found, on the other hand, that it is more desirable to split the prepuce longitudinally on the dorsal aspect with a pair of sharp scissors. Preparatory to this the adhesion of the mucous membrane lining the prepuce to the glans is carefully broken by sweeping the point of the unopened scissors beneath the foreskin. Thus way is made for the introduction of the point of the scissors beneath the prepuce. The skin is first divided and the division of the mucous membrane to a point corresponding to the limit of the division in the skin follows. The mucous membrane is rolled back to the corona and rendered perfectly free. The scissors are now used to trim off the redundant fold of skin on either side of the incision. This is done carefully, while the field of operation is kept free from blood. The redundant roll of skin to the distal side of the frenum is likewise removed in order to avoid the edematous flap, which is often left at this point when enough tissue has not been removed. The skin is now drawn back and carefully inspected in order to deal with any discoverable irregularity in the cut edge. A tape of gauze, a half inch in width and cut so that the edges are frayed, is now applied, securing the roll of mucous membrane in position behind the corona and compressing the bleeding vessels. A tape of about ten inches in length is required in order to admit of several windings. The end of the glans should be left uncovered so that there may be no obstruction to the meatus. It is well to take in, however, the area just beneath the meatus in order to compress the severed frenal artery. One of the greatest safeguards against hemorrhage is to be found in using a coarse-meshed gauze cut with frayed edges in order that it may take up the blood and favor clotting. Over the gauze tape a dry gauze pad is placed and the napkin applied. The wrapping should be changed on the following day and daily thereafter. Otherwise the gauze, which becomes moistened by urine, may cause excoriation. After the second day, instead of the dry gauze, or that moistened by a mild solution of bichlorid or by boric acid solution, a gauze dressing thoroughly spread with vaseline should be applied. This will prevent adhesions of the dressing to the granulations. Should such adhesion occur it would lead to sloughing at the point of adhesion and consequently delayed healing. It is unusual for the swelling to persist after the second or third day.

The indications for the use of sutures in the usual procedure are the coaptation of the skin and mucous membrane and the prevention of hemorrhage. By the use of gauze wrapping the skin and mucous membrane are kept in place, while rapid granulation is favored by the even pressure of the dressing. The bleeding which results from circumcision in the newborn is usually slight, and a moderately firm gauze wrapping, when properly applied, is sufficient to control it. Thus the indications which suggest the use of sutures are fully met by the gauze wrapping. The chance of local infection by the irritation of the sutures when in place is also obviated by the more or less complete protection offered by the gauze.

The objection may be raised that this method is unsurgical, in that we are trusting to an insecure pressure to control hemorrhage and are substituting for sutures a displaceable dressing. These objections may hold in instances where the gauze tape is improperly applied, but only in such instances. Even the apparent unneatness of the dressing is not a valid ground for condemning it, as when the tape is properly cut and evenly applied, especially if it is applied after being moistened, its bulk may be kept within such limits as to make it a neat appearing dressing. If the tape is moistened it usually remains for twenty-four hours without being displaced, but in order to secure it the end of the gauze tape may be split and the two ends thus formed may be lightly tied, as in a finger bandage.

DISCUSSION.

DR. COTTON.—I believe I haven't circumcised a baby in eight or nine years, but earlier in our practice it was the fad to circumcise all male babies that would allow it. Twenty-five years ago I was invited to a ritualistic circumcision and I have attended a number since. That was the first operation I ever saw performed by a Jewish Rabbi and he did more circum-

WILSON : *A Simple Method of Circumcision.*   83

cisions than any other Rabbi in Chicago. I found that he met
with almost uniformly good results. The method was very much
like that described by the essayist. He seized the prepuce with
the thumb and finger, placed over it a little shield made from a
silver half dollar that someone had given him with a slit extending two-thirds the way through it. With the scalpel a downward
sweep was made along this shield, amputating the prepuce. He
then laid the shield aside and, taking the two sides of the cut surface between his fingers and thumbs, he retracted the mucous
lining with the ring fingers, holding the integument tightly. A
little alum water was then applied and a little tape wrapped
around to retain in position the reduplicated tissue. That was
wet with alum water and then a piece of cloth or gauze with a
hole in the middle was applied in such a way as to hold this dressing in place. There was no such thing as sutures, and the cases all
did well. I immediately adopted the method, using a little surgeon's
adhesive tissue. I never saw a case fail to do well in any child
too young to interfere with the dressings with his hands. I do
not, however, recommend the operation as I used to.

DR. WILSON (closing discussion).—The operation may be
carried out with the greatest simplicity by using a pair of surgeon's scissors. The advisability of using the knife is debatable.
I had a very disagreeable experience which led to my adopting
the scissors. Unfortunately, I was using a sharp scalpel, and
just as I made the incision the nurse's attention was diverted and
she neglected to hold the child's legs, which were brought suddenly and forcibly together and the point of the scalpel severed
the left femoral artery. Fortunately, the circumcision was
completed, as I was able to enlarge the incision over the femoral
artery, introducing forceps and catching the proximal end of the
vessel and afterward ligating. It was that experience that induced me to use the more simple method.

CONGENITAL HYPERTROPHIC STENOSIS OF THE PYLORUS IN AN INFANT.—REPORT OF A CASE.

BY JOHN DORNING, M.D.,

New York.

The following case of congenital hypertrophic stenosis of the pylorus is reported merely because it presents the typical clinical features of this now generally recognized disorder and hence may, with propriety, be added to the growing list of recorded cases of this interesting malady.

On May 29, 1905, I saw, in consultation with Dr. M. E. O'Donovan, of New York, Baby McG., seven weeks old, whose history is as follows: The baby was healthy and well developed at birth and weighed between nine and ten pounds. He had vomited since birth, usually after each nursing. On several occasions he did not vomit for a half day, but would afterward regurgitate a large quantity of sour material. He generally smelled sour. On the supposition that the maternal milk was the cause of the stomach disturbance, artificial feeding, consisting of the various infant foods, gruels and milk combinations, was substituted. For five days prior to my visit there had been less vomiting than usual. During these days the food was composed of arrowroot, 1 teaspoonful; whole milk, 3 teaspoonfuls, and hot water, 6 ounces, alternating with a weak solution of gelatin in water. During the past four weeks the vomited matter has been mixed with mucus. He never vomited bile. The stools have always been green, but there has never been any diarrhea. There has been progressive loss of flesh and increasing weakness.

Examination showed a very pale and greatly emaciated baby. The skin of face wrinkled and expression apathetic. The epigastrium was slightly distended. At short intervals a peristaltic wave, from left to right, was observed in the epigastrium. The abdomen was soft and there was no distention or muscular resistance. On deep palpation a nodule, about the size of a large bean, was felt in the epigastric region, just to the right of the median line. Examination of the chest was negative. With such a history and physical signs it was clearly a case of congenital hypertrophic stenosis of the pylorus. An operation was advised and emphatically declined. I then suggested irrigation of the stomach and a food mixture of whey, dextrinized gruel and cream. I did not again see the child, but the subsequent history obtained from the doctor was, that he was not permitted to irrigate the stomach; that the food suggested seemed to agree and was for the most part retained. There had been much less vomiting since our consultation. The child seemed to improve for about ten days and then gradually failed and died on June 16th. An autopsy was not allowed.

While hypertrophic stenosis of the pylorus in infancy is a condition not frequently observed, still, in view of the many cases reported during the past ten or twelve years, it cannot be said to be a rare affection. It is well, however, to keep the malady in mind, so that an early diagnosis may be made and the little patient given the benefit of an operation before his vitality becomes exhausted. For with our present knowledge of this condition an operation is really the only measure that offers any hope of recovery in the majority of cases.

In an article, illustrated with a photo-micrograph of a section of an hypertrophied pylorus, published by the writer in the ARCHIVES OF PEDIATRICS, 1904, may be found a bibliography of the subject.

CONGENITAL MALFORMATION OF THE ESOPHAGUS WITH THE REPORT OF A CASE.*

BY J. P. CROZER GRIFFITH, M.D.,

Clinical Professor of Diseases of Children in the University of Pennsylvania,

AND

R. S. LAVENSON, M.D.,

Assistant Physician to the Philadelphia Hospital; Assistant Pathologist to the Hospital of the University of Pennsylvania, Philadelphia.

Although malformations of the esophagus have been reported with considerable frequency on account of the striking symptoms presented, they are, in fact, comparatively uncommon. Careful study of the matter has been made by Mackenzie, Kraus, Marsh, Phillips and others. Mackenzie could collect but 63 cases, and Dickie, writing in 1906, found but 13 additional ones. He fails, however, to mention these by name. The most valuable contribution of recent date is that of Happich, in which, as well as in Mackenzie's text-book, will be found the bibliography for reported cases not specifically mentioned by us.

Malformations may be of various forms. Ignoring bronchial clefts which belong rather to another category, these may be:—

(1) *Total Absence of the Esophagus.*—This is a very rare condition associated generally with other serious malformations, such as seen in acephalous monsters with defects in the thoracic and abdominal viscera. Happich collects 7 cases of this anomaly, viz., those of Sonderland, Tiedemann, Cooper, Mondière, Lozach, Heath, and Mackenzie. Kraus adds none to the list; and we have found no records elsewhere.

(2) *Partial or Complete Doubling of the Esophagus.*—This also is an extremely rare disorder, there being in Happich's list only the 2 cases reported by Blasius. To this we may add the case of Kathe, published in 1907, in which a narrow supplemental lumen appeared to exist in the wall of the tube.

(3) *Tracheoesophageal Fistula without other Lesion of the Esophagus.*—Like the others this is also very rarely seen. Happich quotes but 4 cases, those of Pinard Tarnier, Richter, and von de Water; and reference to the original communication shows that the reports of Pinard and Tarnier were upon the same case, so that the number is actually but 3. Kraus mentions the 3 cases of Vrolick, Lamb and Eppinger.

(4) *Stenosis.*—The cause of this may be either a fold of

---

* From the Children's Medical Ward and the Pepper Clinical Laboratory of the University of Pennsylvania.

mucous membrane, as is the cases of Rossi, Tenon, Kraus, and others, or a narrowing involving the entire wall of the esophagus, as in the case of Hirschsprung. In certain instances of stenosis recorded, viz., those of Home, Cassan and Berg, and Follin, it is far from sure that the condition was congenital in origin. Very probably carcinoma may have been the cause. Omitting these we have found the records of but 20 cases, viz., Rossi, Tenon, Bauernfeind, Gianella, Siegert, Worthington, Brenner, Zenker, Mayer, Hirschsprung, Schneider, Cruveilhier, Blasius, Fagge, Wilks, Turner, Crary, Baillie, Wadstein, and Demme.

(5) *Congenital Dilatation.*—This is limited to the portion of the esophagus just above the diaphragm. The condition was first described by Arnold and by Luschka, the latter of whom applied to it the appropriate term "Vormagen." The case described by Rotch appears to be a very typical instance. The condition may lead to a secondary diffuse dilatation involving the entire length of the esophagus. Although Vigot, it is true, described funnel-shaped diverticula arising from the anterior wall of the esophagus, it is doubtful whether these are ever really congenital. It is claimed by some that the foundation for the development of pulsion diverticula is laid in a congenital weakness of the muscular elements of the esophageal wall.

(6) *Obliteration of the Esophagus in only a Portion of its Extent, Unaccompanied by Fistula.*—This, too, is very uncommon. There are several varieties. Only the upper portion of the esophagus may be normal, the position and extent of the lower obliterated fragment varying with the case. This was true in the cases of Brodie, Durston, Schoeller and others, that of Durston being the first case of congenital malformation of the esophagus recorded by anyone. In other instances both upper and lower fragments of the esophagus are patulous, and a more or less distinct muscular or connective tissue cord or band united them, as in the cases of Marsh, Weill and Pehu, Steel, and Shattock. Whatever the form, the degree of preservation of the obliterated portion is subject to great variation. In some cases the esophagus is described as entirely absent. In others, the cord-like character was distinctly present. In some, as in the case of Phillips, there seemed to be an absolute disappearance of the intervening portion of the esophagus, but microscopical examination showed remains of the esophageal tissues. In all, of course, the lumen of the affected portion was completely obliterated. The term "obliteration" is, indeed, only used here to describe the condition of the *lumen*, whatever the state of the walls might be.

It is questionable whether in any of the reported cases the tissues of the obliterated portion of the esophagus have been entirely wanting. The matter could be settled in any instance only by careful, and often microscopical, study of the posterior wall of the trachea, since the tissues of the esophagus are firmly attached to this region and often apparently lost in it.

Happich has collected only 11 cases of this partial obliteration of the esophagus without fistula, viz., those of Marrigues, Lallemand, Brodie, Durston, Röderer, Toujan, Lichty, Shattock, van Cruyk, Weill and Pehu and Marsh.

We may add the case of Steel, 3 cases of Kraus and the 2 cases recently reported by Phillips, to one of which we have just referred.

(7) *Obliteration of a Portion of the Esophagus with Tracheoesophageal (or Bronchoesophageal) Fistula.*—This is by far the most frequent malformation found. Of Mackenzie's 63 cases of esophageal malformations, 43 were of this nature, and Happich has tabulated carefully 59. Detailed enumeration of these may be obtained in the bibliography of these two writers. We have found published in the last six years 14 additional instances, 12 of them since the appearance of Happich's monograph. These are, viz., cases of Kirmisson, Renault, Villemin, Patron, Keith and Spicer (4 cases), Dickie, Guyot, Fischer, Spicer, and Giffhorn (2 cases). Another case very briefly reported by Guillemet probably belongs to this category. In addition, there are 2 cases published by Dam and by Wunsch respectively, in which there was no autopsy made, but in which an obstruction was discovered by the use of a sound, and which possibly belong here also.

Malformations elsewhere in the body are very liable to occur in combination with this defect (28 of Happich's 59 cases), as, in fact, with congenital defect of the esophagus of whatever nature. The occlusion of the esophagus may be very short, or may exist in the form of a fibrous cord which is either quite evident or almost indistinguishable, and which may or may not contain distinct evidences of muscular fibre. The esophagus throughout its extent is generally firmly adherent to the trachea, and the obliterated portion especially so, or even almost indistinguishable from the posterior tracheal wall. The obliteration is almost always situated at or a little above the bifurcation of the trachea. When it is of very short length the two fragments of the esophagus frequently appear to overlap each other. The upper fragment of the esophagus is generally dilated, with its walls hypertrophied. It is usually rather funnel-form than cylindrical, and ends blindly at the point of obstruction. As a rule, the lower fragment is of normal calibre for some distance above the stomach, and then gradually tapers in an upward direction, ending in a fistula into the trachea. It is noticeable that the fistula is always in the lower fragment. The only exception recorded is that of Fischer, in which, in addition to the usual fistula in the lower portion, there was also a very minute opening into the trachea from the upper fragment of the esophagus. The fistula is usually slit-like in form and enters the trachea oftenest shortly above the bifurcation; less often just at the position of the bifurcation. Fistula into the bronchus is extremely rare. Mackenzie found it recorded but 3 times and Happich adds none to the list. We have found 1 additional case reported by Kirmisson in 1904.

The case which we desire to place on record belongs to the class of obliteration with tracheoesophageal fistula. The notes are as follows:—

Joseph Dorland, nine days old, was admitted to the Hospital of the University of Pennsylvania, December 7, 1907. The parents were living and well. Five other healthy children had been born. The patient was a full term infant, delivered with forceps after a somewhat difficult labor. Since birth he had never been able to swallow. After taking the breast for a moment he would become cyanotic, struggle as though strangling, and then eject milk and usually a large amount of mucus from the nose and mouth. Apparently no nourishment whatever passed into the stomach. There was no vomiting except after nursing. Very small bowel movements occurred about twice a day. There had been jaundice since birth. Examination on admission showed an extremely emaciated child. Attempts to feed it were at once followed by the regurgitation and strangling described. The child died a few hours after admission.

The autopsy revealed the body of a well-formed, emaciated infant. The features of interest in the examination of the internal organs were limited to the esophagus and the adjacent parts. The pharyngeal portion of the esophagus was slightly dilated, but otherwise normal to 4 cm. below the upper level of the larynx, where it terminated abruptly. The inferior portion was normal from the stomach upward to within a short distance of the termination of the upper fragment, where the lumen became narrower and, inclining slightly anteriorly, opened by a slit-like orifice into the trachea slightly above the level of the lower end of the upper fragment. The accompanying drawing (Fig. 1) gives a diagrammatic representation of the condition which the esophagus exhibited. An examination of the rest of the thoracic and abdominal viscera revealed no additional malformations or other pathological features.

Pathology.—Malformations of the esophagus doubtless arise in various ways, but in no form is the pathological explanation very certain and in some very unsatisfactory :—

Entire absence of the esophagus can occasion no surprise, as it is seen only in conjunction with other so extensive and serious malformations.

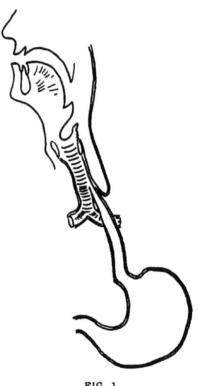

The occurrence of the *complete absence of only a portion* of the esophagus is very problematical. As already stated, some traces of esophageal tissue probably always remain. No satisfactory explanation for it seems to offer. Kleb's theory is that in the development of the respiratory organs from the gut-tract too much tissue was consumed at the expense of the esophagus, this resulting in a localized complete disappearance of the tissues of the latter. The cases in which more or less of the esophageal wall is evidently present in the

FIG. 1.

form of a cord or band Kraus explains as resulting from a form of pressure-atrophy. He has observed 3 instances of this anomaly, in all of which there was compression of the obliterated area by an anomalous vessel. In 2 of them this was the right subclavian artery, which arose as an independent vessel and as the last branch from the arch of the aorta, which lay behind the esophagus.

Simple fistula without other lesion is apparently the result of the persistence of the embryological communication between the primitive gut-tract and the cervical portion of the air passages. As this embryonic communication exists between the air passages at or just above the bifurcation of the trachea and the corresponding portion of the esophagus, the resulting fistula is practically always at this point.

Congenital *stenotic conditions* probably depend upon accidental changes in some part of the esophageal wall.

The greatest interest attaches to the pathology of the most common anomaly, *i.e.*, *obliteration of the esophagus with tracheo-esophageal fistula,* and the questions naturally arise, Why fistula is so usually combined with obliteration? Why the obliteration is always close to the position of the bifurcation of the trachea? and Why the fistula is always found in the lower fragment of the in-

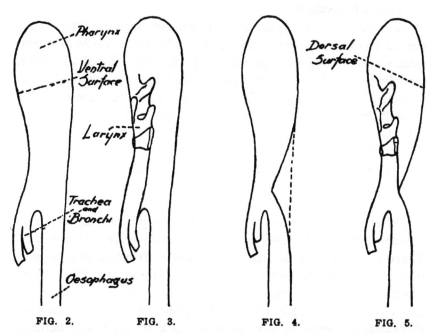

FIG. 2.　　　FIG. 3.　　　FIG. 4.　　　FIG. 5.

Illustrating production of congenital obliteration of esophagus with formation of tracheoesophageal fistula. After Shattock.

terrupted esophagus? The most satisfactory explanation of the mode of formation of this abnormality is that proposed by Shattock. According to his view, at the time when the pouch from which the lower air passages develop is formed from the anterior wall of the stomadeum, the posterior wall occasionally participates in the process sufficiently to be drawn forward, thus narrowing the lumen. When, subsequently, the lateral pouching for the formation of the larynx develops from the stomadeum just above this region, so much of the already narrowed lumen is consumed that the communication between the upper and lower portions of the esophagus is cut off and the lower fragment is left communicating with the air passages.

The process can be probably better understood by a glance at the accompanying diagrammatic illustrations taken from Shattock's article. Fig. 2 represents the normal development of the lower air passages from the diverticulum on the anterior wall of the stomadeum, and Fig. 3 the development, from its pharyngeal extremity, of the larynx and upper part of the trachea. In Fig. 4 the abnormal kink in the posterior wall is seen opposite the diverticulum, and Fig. 5 illustrates the subsequent development of the larynx and upper part of the trachea dividing the esophagus into two portions, the lower of which remains in communication with the air passages.

Symptoms.—The symptoms of stenosis seen in infancy are similar to those observed later in life. The same is true of dilatation, whether congenital or following stenosis. We shall confine ourselves, therefore, to the symptomatology of congenital obliteration of the esophagus. The children with this condition may be well developed, but are often the subjects of congenital asthenia. Other malformations are very frequently present. From the time of birth there seems to be an unusual amount of mucus constantly expelled from the mouth. This is due to the fact that the oral secretion cannot pass into the stomach as it does in the case of healthy children. No food whatever can enter the stomach, and efforts at swallowing are attended by a prompt regurgitation through the mouth and nose of the food mixed with mucus. There are produced in this way violent suffocative attacks with severe cyanosis. Attempts at passing a catheter into the esophagus meet with the obstruction. Death takes place generally in the first week, exceptionally later, and depends in part upon the constitutional asthenia, in part upon the lack of food, and perhaps still more, as Happich points out, upon the drying of the tissues through lack of water.

Treatment.—This is entirely discouraging. Cases of stenosis have recovered, but all instances of complete obstruction have died. The weakness of the child and its early age make operative interference a questionable procedure. Yet gastrostomy offers the only hope. This operation was first done in the case of Steel, and has been performed since then in those of Hoffmann, Happich, Villemin, Kirmisson, and Dickie. The child should be kept on its side to allow the mucus to flow from the mouth. It may be fed through the gastric fistula. Should it recover, an effort may later be made to repair the esophagus by a lateral operation in the neck. This indeed was attempted unsuccessfully in Hoffmann's case as a primary operation, and gastrostomy resorted to later.

(Discussion on page 99.)

BIBLIOGRAPHY.

Arnold. Untersuch. im Gebiete f. Anat. u. Phys., 1888, 211.
Baillie. Traité d'Anat. path., 1808, 98.
Bauerfeind. Inaug. Dissert. München, 1893.
Blasius. Ger. observata anatom. pract. in homine, Ludg. Batav. et Amsterlod., 1674, Tab. XV., Fig. 6.
Blasius. Ger. observata medica rariora. Amst., 1677, Pars IV., Tab. VI., Fig. 2.
Brenner. Beitr. z. Chir.; Billroth-Festschrift, 1892.
Brodie. Biblioteca medica, 1810, 881.
Cannan and Berg. Arch. gen. de Med., 1826, 79.
Cooper. Traité d'Anat. path., I., 475.
Crary. Quoted by Kraus (q. v.).
Cruveilhier. Path. Anat. de Corps humaine, 1835-42, T. II., L. XXXVIII., pl. VI.
    "   Traité path, gen., 1849, T. II., 232.
Van Cruyk. Bull. Soc. med. d'emulation de Paris, 1824, 23.
Dam. Presse med. beige, 1906. LVIII., 589.
Demme. Quoted by Korman. 7. Berichte u. d. Jennersche Kinderspital z. Bern.
Dickie. Brit. Journ. Child. Dis., 1906, III., 411.
Durston. Collect. Academ. Part. etrang., 1670, T. II.. 283.
Eppinger. Path. Anat. d. Larynx u. d. Trachea, 1880, 252.
Fagge. Guys Hosp. Rep., 1872, XVII., 413.
Fisher. Zentralbl. f. path. Anat., 1905, XVI., 1.
Follin. Bull. della Soc. med., 1853, XIX., 267.
Gianella. De Dysphagia. Instit. med. pract., IV., 292.
Giffhorn. Virch. Archiv., 1908, CXCII., H. 1, 112.
Guillemet. Gaz. med. de Nantes, 1906, 2s., XXIV., 576.
Guyot. Bull. et Mem., Soc. Anat. de Paris, 1907, LXXXII., 384.
Happich. Inaug. Dissert. Marburg, 1905.
Heath. Lond. Med. Gaz., 1840, XXVI., 542.
Hirschsprung. Inaug. Dissert. Kopenhagen, 1861.
    "   Hospitals Tidende, 1895. No. 42.
Hoffmann. Inaug. Dissert. Greifsw., 1899.
Home. Bibliotheca medica., T. 8. 260.
Kathe. Virchows Archiv., 1907, CXC., 78.
Keith and Spicer. Journ. Anat. and Physiol., 1906, XLI., 52.
Kirmisson. Bull. et Mem. de la Soc. de Chir. de Paris, 1904, N. S. XXX., 745.
Klebs. Qt. by Eppinger (q. v.).
Kraus. Nothnagel's Spec. Path. u. Therap., 1902, VXI., 93.
Lallemand. Thèse de Paris, 1816.
Lamb. Phila. Med. Times, 1873, 705.
Lichty. Journ. Amer. Med. Assoc., 1896, Aug.
Lozach. Journal Universel.,1816, III., 187.
Luschka. Virchows Archiv., 1848, XLVII., 178.
Mackenzie. Diseases of the Throat and Nose, 1880, II.. 220.
Marrigues. Mem. de math. Préc., T. IV., 123. (Quoted by Happich.)
Marsh. Amer. Journ. Med. Sci., 1902, CXXIV., 304.
Mayer. Amer. Journ. Med. Sci., 1893, CVI., 567.
Mondiere. Hufeland's Journ., 1820, Aug. L. 2, 133.
Patron. Gaz. Med. de Nantes, 1906, 2s., XXIV., 573.
Phillips. ARCH. OF PEDIAT., 1908, April, 267.
Pinard. Bull. Soc. Anat., 1873, XLVIII., 682 ; 685.
Renault. Bull. Med., 1904, XVIII., 479.
Richter. Inaug. Dissert., Leipzig, 1792.
Röderer. Fetus parasitici descr. in comm. Soc. reg. Goetting; ad Annal., 1754, T., III., 113.
Rossi. Mem. dell'Acad. d. Sci. di Torino, 1826, XXX., I., 155.
Rotch. Pediatrics, 1901, 769.
Schneider. Inaug. Dissert. Königsberg, 1900.
Schoeller. Neue Zeitsch. f. Geburtsk., 1838, VI., 264.
Shattock. Trans. Path. Soc., London, 1890, XLI., 87.
Siegert. Inaug. Dissert. Halle, 1856.
Sonderland. Harless Rheinische Jahrbücher, I., St. 22, 198.
Spicer. Lancet, 1907, I., 157.
Steel. Lancet, 1888, II., 764.
Tarnier. Gaz. Med. de Paris, 1866, No. 29.
    "   Gaz. des Hôp., 1873, No. 173.
Tenon. La med. eclairee parles Sciences, phys., T. I., 301.
Tiedemann. Anatomie kopfloser Missgeburten (Quoted by Schoeller.)
Toujau. Ann. de gyn. et obstet., 1892, XXXVIII., 38.
Turner. Quoted by Kraus.
Vigot. Assoc. franc. pour l'avancement des Sci., 23 Sess. Carn., 1894, Confer. de Paris, 206. (Quoted by Kraus.)
Villemin. Bull. de la Soc. de Ped. de Paris, 1904, VI., 228.
Vrolik. Tabulæ ad illustrandam embryogenesis. Amst., 1849, Tab. 89, Fig. 2.
Wadstein. Nord. med. Ark., 1894, XXIV., No. 21, 25.
Von de Water. Inaug. Dissert., Leyden, 1857.
Weill and Pehu. Lyon med., 1900, No. 9.
Wilks. Path. Transac., London, 1866, XVII., 138.
Worthington. Med.-Chir. Transac., 1847, XXX., 199.
Wunsch. Med. Klinik., Berlin, 1907, III., 389.
Zenker. Zenker u. Ziemssen, Oesophagus Krankh., Leipzig, 1874, 19.

A CASE OF SPASMODIC STRICTURE OF THE ESOPHAGUS.

BY SAMUEL S. ADAMS, M.D.,

Washington, D. C.

On the afternoon of February 17, 1907, I was called to attend A. X., aged six months, white, female, born in this city. The following history was obtained:—

Parents living and in good health. No history of neurosis in either. This their only child. The child's birth was normal and she was nursed by the mother for one week, when various "infant foods" and "milk mixtures" were "tried," but she did not get on very well and was troubled with "sour stomach." Has had no "serious illness."

About six weeks ago she began to have difficulty in swallowing food. At times the slightest amount would be returned, accompanied by considerable mucus, for several feedings, and then she would retain all food given for several days until "another spell occurred." During the periods of returning the food it did not seem to come from the stomach as it was not completely swallowed. She never vomited blood. Mother declares long naps or exposure to drafts were invariably associated with the attacks. Parents were certain the infant had never swallowed any caustic, or foreign body; nor had she ever been given any sleep-producing drugs.

The attacks have become less frequent and less severe, the last being on the 13th of this month. She "does not seem to have lost any weight," although she weighed 9 pounds at birth and at present weighs 8 pounds 5½ ounces. About two weeks ago her feet and ankles began to swell, but this soon disappeared. Has been more or less constipated since birth.

The last feeding was at 1 A.M. to-day.

General Examination.—Expression anxious; of average height; weight below average; nutrition poor; anterior fontanel very large and depressed; veins of the forehead distended; intelligence average; no teeth; restless; no eruption; temperature normal.

The cutaneous, muscular and osseous systems apparently normal. Slight enlargement of the inguinal glands. Lips and gums dry, tongue slightly coated; abdomen slightly distended; constipated.

Considerable mucus in nose and mouth; otherwise respiratory system normal.

Circulatory system normal.

Genitourinary system normal.

Infant fretful and cries a great deal, but there is no history of convulsions or other nervous manifestation.

There is no evidence of rickets; nor could any symptom of laryngismus stridulus be elicited.

It was now seventeen hours since the child had swallowed food, and, as she was both thirsty and hungry, I directed the father to give her some cool water. She swallowed two teaspoonfuls and then refused to take any more. In two or three minutes she began to gulp and gag; at first the water came back into the mouth and was again swallowed; then water and mucus; and finally, after probably a dozen attempts to get it down, the water and as much mucus was ejected.

I was sure of an obstruction in the esophagus, and expressed the belief that it was spasmodic in character. At my suggestion the infant was taken to the Children's Hospital, D. C., at 9 P.M., and was seen by Dr. J. R. Wellington, the surgeon, and me.

Dr. Wellington tried to pass an ordinary sized feeding tube, but it met an obstruction just above the stomach which it would not pass; a smaller catheter would not pass; finally a No. 10 French catheter with stylet was gently pushed by the obstruction into the stomach. Through this was passed four ounces of a suitable milk mixture, which was retained.

During the night nutritive enemata were given, but were not well retained.

February 18th.—She had rather a restless night; vomited a small quantity of bilious-looking fluid, after which she felt better. She was placed on the table for the purpose of having the tube passed, when Dr. Wellington directed the nurse to give her some milk that he might see how she acted or swallowed. He was greatly amazed to see that she swallowed and retained the full amount of nourishment, and went to sleep.

This sudden improvement aroused a suspicion that some foreign body might have been pushed into the stomach the previous night, but nothing unusual was detected by the X-ray.

The infant took eagerly and retained its nourishment for the next four days and gained in weight.

February 22d.—Dr. Wellington passed with some difficulty a No. 18 soft rubber French catheter. The doctor thought that if he passed the catheter quickly it met with less resistance than when he passed it slowly.

February 23d.—She was taken away by her parents and was in much better condition than when admitted.

May 30, 1907.—I have indirectly followed the history of this case, which has continued to have the attacks, but less frequently than before the tube was passed. A few days ago I learned from the father that she was now having attacks about every two weeks and that they only lasted an hour or two. He said his wife thought that the infant would overcome the difficulty in swallowing when she would startle her by a shout or a clap of the hands.

May 4, 1908.—During the past year I did not attend the child but frequently saw her in the carriage. On inquiry from time to time I learned that there was not much improvement, although she grew slowly and had learned to walk and talk. To-day, as I was about to enter the Georgetown University Hospital, the father stopped me and wanted me to do something to relieve his child, as she had not swallowed a thing for twenty-four hours and had cried most of that time, so that her mother and himself were about worn out. He pulled from his pocket several metallic sounds and suggested that they could be used. I declined to treat the child, but advised him to consult a surgeon at once.

May 5, 1908.—About 6 P.M. the father telephoned to me that his child was very ill; that the surgeon had passed the sounds that morning; that she had "cried with pain" all day; and that she now had considerable fever. I told him to ask one of the internes to see her and report to me. Two hours later he urged me to see the child and I did so. Her temperature in the rectum was 104° F., pulse 170 and respiration 70 and labored. I made a diagnosis of bronchopneumonia, but was accused of trying to shield the surgeon. At midnight the father telephoned that she was worse, so I requested a physician in the neighborhood to see her, but she was dead when he reached the house. The next day I signed the death certificate, giving bronchopneumonia as the cause of death, but, owing to the abuse heaped upon the surgeon and myself by the father, I withdrew the certificate and reported the case to the coroner. Following is his report:—

May 6, 1907.—12 M. White, female, aged one year nine months; weight, 22 pounds. (?)

Previous History.—Symptoms of stenosis of the esophagus. Body had been embalmed. General nutrition good. Slight pallor. Brain not opened. Lungs: Several areas of red hepatization throughout the left lung, lobular condition. Several bronchial glands markedly enlarged. Hypostasis posteriorly on both lungs. Heart, spleen, kidneys, urine, liver, gall-bladder, pancreas, stomach, intestines and genital organs normal.

Esophagus: five inches above cardiac orifice of stomach marked narrowing (circular) of the tube; appeared as an induration between the walls, markedly uniform. The condition of induration extended upwards one inch. Immediately adjacent to the induration on the left side was found a bronchial gland about the size of a chestnut which was pressing inwards upon the tube.

Microscopically the gland appeared to be tuberculous. At the beginning of the normal tube, above stenosis on left side, a well-defined diverticulum was noted, which was about the size of a No. 10 bird-shot. A perforation into the mediastinum, with a blood-clot, was found. Just below stenosis area on anterior wall two other diverticula were noted, about the size of the one described, their walls being very thin, consisting only of the external coat.

The specimen was given to the pathologist, who pronounced the glands to be tuberculous, but repeated efforts to get a complete report from him have failed.

As neither food nor foreign substance was found in the mediastinum, the perforation had nothing to do with the child's death. On the contrary, I believe the pneumonia, the cause of death, was due to the inspiration of food and antedated the passage of the sounds on the morning of her death. This opinion is strengthened by the fact that on the preceding day her father reported her condition as being serious and, from a casual observation, his statement was accepted.

Dr. Prentiss Willson examined the literature at the Library of the Surgeon-General's Office and could only find 1 case that resembled the above. The following is an abstract of an article by Méry* on "Spasms of the Alimentary Canal in Nurslings."

These spasmodic conditions may attack the pylorus, esophagus or cardia. Sometimes the cause is intoxication, in other cases

---

* *Rev. gen. de clin. et de Therap.*, Paris, 1906, XX. 51-53.

nothing but a nervous element can be given as the etiologic factor. After mentioning 3 cases of pyloric spasm, he continues as follows: Instead of attacking the pylorus, the spasms may attack the cardia or esophagus. *This is exceptional.* Comby, in his "Treatise on the Diseases of Childhood," does not mention the occurrence of esophagism before the seventh to tenth years. The case now to be described is that of a little girl ten months of age, breast-fed for the first three months. No trace of nervous manifestations in the parents. In the fourth month, without previous digestive infection, the child was taken with an attack of asphyxia of great severity, nutrition became bad and during the interval of five months, from September to February, the increase in weight was only 500 grams. Three developed attacks of forcible vomiting, following *immediately* the ingestion of fluids, accompanied by slight laryngeal stridor and some hiccough. During this time the child slept well, the stools were normal and she had no fever. Glairy mucus streaked with blood, was occasionally rejected with the milk. Various diets and therapeutic agents were tried without avail.

After giving the child milk of bismuth, radioscopy showed a black mass above the stomach, and in about thirty seconds part of it could be seen entering the stomach, and the remainder would be rejected. By introducing a rigid sound gavage was attempted, but the stomach contracted so on the eye of the instrument that it was necessary to use a syringe and considerable force to inject the milk. The child was isolated, taken from its mother, and put under the care of a nurse. It soon developed a general edema, spasms of the glottis and convulsive twitchings of the right side attributed to edema of the brain, but ultimately recovered. Méry considers the esophageal spasm as possibly attributable to the ingestion of air while sucking the thumb, a habit to which the child was addicted. He thought that the attacks of esophageal spasm decreased in frequency when the infant was prevented from sucking its thumb.

Although Méry's case resembles in some respects my own nevertheless, one must conclude, from his description of it, that it is a good picture of laryngismus stridulus in a rachitic infant.

The infant in my case used the cotton-plugged nipple as a pacifier and the father says that I suggested that it might have had something to do with the attacks, so they stopped using it.

1 Dupont Circle.

DISCUSSION OF PAPERS OF DR. GRIFFITH AND DR. ADAMS.

AUGUSTUS CAILLÉ, M.D., New York.—In connection with Dr. Adams' case, I would report a somewhat similar one; a lad of ten, who is now under my observation, the son of a physician, has had a spasmodic stricture for five years. Five years ago careful examination elicited the fact that there was no diverticulum—it was purely spasmodic. The stricture came on gradually and the inability to swallow was such that the boy was moribund from starvation. There was no difficulty in introducing the usual calibre tube and he was fed in that way. After some time he became able to swallow and was taken home. The father is still compelled once or twice a week to use the tube for feeding him.

This lad had hydrocephalus in his infancy and I imagine the irritation is of central origin, and I doubt if it will ever get entirely well.

In this connection I would sound a note of warning regarding the examination of the esophagus by means of the sound or esophagoscope. I have recently seen a young girl, who had some difficulty in swallowing, who was examined with the esophagoscope by an expert stomach specialist. He ran the instrument into the left pleural cavity, a pneumothorax developed and she was dead in two days.

C. P. PUTNAM, M.D., Boston.—I should like to mention a case similar to Dr. Griffith's; a boy twelve days old, with the history of not having swallowed anything since birth, was brought to the Massachusetts Infant Asylum. A solid obstruction having been found four inches from inside the lips, a gastrostomy was performed successfully by Dr. J. S. Stone. The baby rallied well after the operation and received a little milk with a tube through the wound. The stomach had plainly been empty up to that time. Doubt was thrown upon the diagnosis of obstructed esophagus when next day the baby vomited some milk, but this was explained by the autopsy. On the second day it failed and died.

The autopsy by Dr. Robertson showed that the esophagus ended in a blind pouch a little above the bifurcation of the trachea. The milk introduced into the stomach had been vomited up through the trachea. The child had some consolidation in the bases of both lungs.

THOMAS MORGAN ROTCH, M.D., Boston.—This opens up a rather important point in regard to the differential diagnosis in these cases, especially since we have had in late years much added information in regard to pyloric stenosis. Some of these cases of constriction of the esophagus simulate very closely pyloric stenosis. It is rather curious that they are almost identical so far as the rational signs are concerned. The food will sometimes be kept down for a day or forty-eight hours and then vomited. There is danger in passing the sound because sometimes at the lower part of the esophagus there is a thinning of the wall in these cases. I have had a careful autopsy made on one where there was congenital stenosis just at the entrance to the stomach and above that a ballooning of the esophagus from stretching. In the lower part of the sac there was a very thin place about 1 cm. in diameter which was about to rupture into the trachea. The least mechanical interference would have ruptured it before death. We know that in a certain number of these cases we do not find anything on physical examination, although our recent examinations, especially with the Roentgen ray, have aided very much. These cases also simulate closely cases of chronic gastric indigestion, so that the greatest care should be used, before employing any other method, to carefully regulate the diet so as to determine whether or not they are cases of indigestion.

A. JACOBI, M.D., New York.—What was the exact site of the constriction in Dr. Griffith's case?

DR. GRIFFITH.—Just above the bifurcation.

DR. JACOBI.—It is that position which gives rise to a great deal of difficulty in the adult. Carcinomata of the esophagus are apt to be found in just that position. The cause, I think, must be looked for in embryonal conditions. It is with the esophagus just as with the rectum; there may be just such overlapping. The parts are formed separately and as a rule will meet one another and so the tube is formed, but in this neighborhood there is always a narrowest part. We find that when we introduce a large sound into the esophagus of a healthy person, there is apt to be some constriction and it must be explained by the nature of its embryonal development. In the rectum we find it more frequently perhaps, so frequently that every one of us may have found such a deformity of the rectum that when you mean to open such an imperforate rectum in a newborn by operation it may happen that you find these parts improperly developed so that the trochar runs into the peritoneal cavity in place of into the upper part of the rectum. It is the seat of predilection for cancer even in late life. Such a case of unsuccessful operation for imperforate rectum I published in the *American Medical Journal* of 1861.

As to the diverticuli they may be explained by something that happens a good many times. The muscular layers of the intestinal tract are not uniformly developed. Defects of these layers are quite common. That is the case in the sigmoid. Diverticuli formed below the constriction must be explained in that way. The muscular layers in these places are incompletely developed. Certain places imperfectly developed are found throughout the whole intestinal tract and the upper part of the apparatus is no exception.

SAMUEL S. ADAMS, M.D., Washington.—I would state that there was no fluid found outside of the esophagus in the surrounding tissue, nor was there anything in the bronchial tubes, and yet I believe the pneumonia was probably the result of inhalation of some of the food that the child had been trying to take.

REPORT OF A CASE OF CONGENITAL HEART DISEASE.—DEFECT OF THE VENTRICULAR SEPTUM AND ABSENCE OF THE PULMONARY ARTERY.—SYMPTOMS OF ANGINA PECTORIS.

BY ALFRED HAND, JR., M.D.

of Philadelphia.

A few unusual features in the clinical symptoms and pathological findings induce me to make the following report. As an introduction I quote from Hochsinger's article on "Congenital Heart Disease" in Pfaundler and Schlossmann's *The Diseases of Children,* in which he states that while pulmonary stenosis is very frequent, comprising three-fifths of all congenital cardiac anomalies, and, with a defective septum, allowing of longer life than other forms of congenital heart disease, yet complete obliteration of the pulmonary artery is rare. If the stenosis occurs early in fetal life, then complete partition of the heart is prevented and those portions of the septum which are normally formed under the aortic valves are usually absent. Other authorities state that septal defects are more common in the anterior muscular part than in the membranous part, which is just below the aortic valves, the so-called undefended space.

My own experience is limited to 2 cases, the first one showing a defect in the muscular part, the second, the case under consideration, having a defect primarily of the membranous, but also involving the muscular portion.

The notes of the case are as follows:—

S. J., male, colored, three years old, was admitted to the Children's Hospital on July 10, 1907, for "spells," which began three months ago, the first occurring in April, one in May, two in June, one daily for the first five days of July, and two daily for the five days before admission. The mother described these spells as something like convulsions, starting with a scream, but without biting of the tongue or falling and bruising himself; the child seemed to have pain during the attacks and the breathing was deep, rapid and noisy; the duration of each attack was about an hour, after which the child would go to sleep. The family and personal history obtained on admission was negative, but it was subsequently learned that the doctor who was present at his birth said that he was a "blue baby."

The notes made by the resident physician, Dr. Vail, on admission were: A fairly well-developed boy; head of fair shape; anterior fontanel open the size of a five-cent piece; eyes and ears normal; throat hyperemic; boy walks properly. Lungs everywhere resonant; large râles at both bases; sounds are rough and friction-like at the left base. The heart is rapid and regular. Abdomen not sunken; liver extends 2 cm. below the ribs; spleen is not palpable. Extremities are negative except that the legs and thighs appear under-developed. Kernig's and Babinski's signs are negative; no ankle clonus; no tache. A convulsive or dyspneic attack occurred on July 11, from 7:45 to 9:40 A.M., with much cyanosis, great relaxation, dyspnea, weak and rapid pulse; the child could be aroused; there were no tonic or clonic movements.

When I saw the patient a few hours later physical examination was negative, except for soft breathing over the base of the right lung posteriorly with slight impairment of percussion-resonance at the angle of the scapula, and also marked dullness over the upper part of the sternum. The idea was therefore entertained of an enlarged thymus with attacks of thymic asthma.

On July 12 there was an attack lasting from 12:30 to 3:45 A.M., with dyspnea, cyanosis and suprasternal recession. Examination later showed the lungs to be perfectly clear, but a striking phenomenon was found in the loudness and clearness of the heart sounds, which were heard all over the precordium, to the right of the sternum and up to the second interspace; the sounds seemed close to the ear of the listener, but there was no murmur to account for the clubbing of the fingers; the apex beat was not displaced, but the cardiac dullness extended nearly one cm. to the right of the right border of the sternum. The possibility of enlarged posterior mediastinal glands pushing the heart forward was considered, but Eustace Smith's sign was negative.

On the following day, July 13, I had my first opportunity of seeing him in an attack; he was lying on the right side with his hands pressed against the precordium; his face bore an expression of pain and there was an audible groan with each expiration, the respirations being slow and labored. On auscultation the air was heard entering the lungs easily, the heart sounds were tumultuous and loud and the precordium heaved with the force of the beats, with which the feebleness of the radial pulse contrasted strongly. The mind seemed perfectly clear. The whole attitude and the symptoms suggested pain connected with the heart, an angina pectoris; so a hypodermic injection of morphin (gr. $^1/_{12}$) was immediately given, and in twenty-five minutes the patient was asleep. In the absence of murmurs, what the pathological cardiac lesion was could only be conjectured beyond a decided hypertrophy, with some degree of dilatation. Although there was no generalized nor local edema, failing compensation was undoubtedly present, as shown by the high hemoglobin count, above the maximum figure of 120 per cent. on the Dare scale, and the high count of the red cells, the figures for which were unfortunately not recorded. The attacks of pain were also looked on as due to an acute dilatation of the different chambers of the heart, more particularly of the auricles following that of the left ventricle, which seemed overworked in a vain attempt to overcome some great resistance to the general circulation.

The attacks were subsequently controlled in the severity of the pain by the use of morphin, a hypodermic at the onset being followed by relief in a few minutes, but the frequency remained the same, and an alarming one occurred on the seventh day after admission, with cessation of respiration for a short time.

Fever was present every day, of an irregular type, the morning temperature being usually normal and the evening showing a rise to 103° or 104°, until the tenth day after admission, when it rose to 107.4° just before death.

At the autopsy, aside from a hypostatic congestion of the lungs and anemic infarcts in the spleen and left kidney, the main interest centered in the thymus, which was decidedly enlarged, and in the heart, which extended 4½ cm. to the right and 6½ cm. to the left of the midsternal line; its dimensions were 9½ cm. long, 7½ cm. wide, and 3 cm. thick, and it weighed 115 grams. Careful search failed to disclose any trace of the pulmonary artery, but there was a great deficiency of the interventricular septum, and the ventricular wall, especially on the left, showed decided hypertrophy. The absence of the pulmonary artery and the appearance of the endocardium explained the absence of murmurs during life and the inability to diagnose the condition.

DISCUSSION.

DR. JACOBI.—The nutrition of the lungs in these cases takes place by dilated bronchial arteries coming from the aorta. They take the place of the ramifications of the pulmonary artery, which is absent or stenosed. Life in such cases may be prolonged, as the writer has said. I published such a case in the ARCHIVES OF PEDIATRICS some ten years ago. The patient was twenty-nine when he died and he died only of very copious pulmonary hemorrhage. I believe that these cases are not very rare, and most of them are diagnosticable, as the writer says. There is a loud systolic murmur in many that extends all over the heart, by no means in all. The fact that the two ventricles are alike is simply the same as we have at birth—then the two *are* alike, normally. The circulation remains fetal, as it were, and the two ventricles remain alike.

MODERN LABORATORY FEEDING AND THE WIDE RANGE OF RESOURCES WHICH IT PROVIDES.

BY THOMAS MORGAN ROTCH, M.D.,

Boston, Mass.

Since the year 1891, when the attention of physicians was first turned to the methods of laboratory feeding, a great deal has been accomplished year by year in perfecting more precise methods of dealing with the nutrition of early life, the object always being kept in view of placing the subject of feeding in as simple and practical a way as possible before the medical profession and the laity. I have thought it worth while, after these seventeen years of careful study of the subject, to present to you what has been accomplished, and what a wide range of resources the modern laboratory methods provide. During the development of the question of percentage feeding, I have frequently been impressed with the difficulties which physicians have told me they met with when they found that they were not able, in some special case, to accomplish by these modern methods the favorable results they said they saw apparently follow the use of the various patent and proprietary foods. Notwithstanding these reports, to which I have always listened attentively and endeavored to explain in some rational way, I cannot but feel that there is nothing, after all, so mysterious in the at times successful use of these foods. The subject essentially deals with the nutrition of the infant as effected by all known food stuffs. The food stuffs which make up practically all possible foods can be classified under three headings—fats, carbohydrates and proteids. Any other substances which are used in concurrence with these food stuffs, such as water, mineral salts, alkalies and ferments, are merely added to facilitate the digestion of the above-mentioned compounds of food. However much, as special students of infant feeding, we may each know regarding the use of these three classes of food stuffs, there is no doubt that physicians, in general, as well as the public who employ these physicians, know very little about the vital .

principles of physiological chemistry, which are so interwoven with the whole question of infant feeding. The majority of physicians, for instance, after having made up their minds that they wish to carry out in their practice the principles which were first enunciated by those who believed in the exact method of feeding provided by the milk laboratories, have continued to prescribe on the same routine lines. They have done this without having taken the trouble to inquire whether the earlier ideas on the subject have changed or improved, or whether through means of the laboratories the latest advances in the physiological chemistry of digestion can practically be made use of in every-day practice, in cases where the infant is fed from laboratory products and by laboratory methods. On the prescriptions which emanate from the laboratories it has, indeed, for many years, been explained how the different classes of proteids can be prescribed and used, but this is about all, with the exception of writing for the various food compounds in percentages, that has been accomplished. I have, therefore, thought that the time had come when, for the convenience of physicians in general, the possibilities of what can be accomplished by a new and more advanced prescription card should be explained. I have also thought that besides writing for the percentages of fat, lactose and proteids, as has heretofore been done, we might go further and introduce, by means of an explanatory prescription blank, various new foods, thus showing the physician not only how to write for each food, or the various combinations of the food stuffs, but also to inform him what this writing of prescriptions really means. In order to do this satisfactorily, we should each one of us understand what possibilities there are in prescriptions. If these possibilities are understood, physicians will soon see that the use of the patent foods is entirely unnecessary, for even granting that success may follow their use, we must allow that none but the three classes of food stuffs above mentioned can be used, and that there is no new or unexplained virtue which they contain. The key to the whole question is that we should first understand what the constituents of these foods are. We should next investigate why, from their own peculiar combinations of food stuffs, the various patent foods are at times apparently superior in their results to the recognized laboratory combinations.

This has already been done, and now all combinations of food can be obtained at the laboratories according to the individual practitioner's preference.

Beginning with the investigation of the fats, although we know it is the quality of the fat, as well as the quantity, which makes its use successful in the feeding of an individual infant, yet the only variation besides the percentage which it is possible to obtain at the present time is by using the cream from different breeds of cows, for it is well known that the quality of the fats differs markedly in different breeds. Thus, if we take as examples the creams from Holsteins and Jerseys, a number of differences can be noted. The emulsion of the fat is finer in the Holstein than in the Jersey; is much less easily disturbed, and is restored much more readily. It has not only been found that the calves of Jersey cows thrive better on the milk of common cows than on that of their own mothers, but that in the feeding of pigs a milk poor in fat has been found to be the best. The question of high or low fats in infant feeding I shall not enter into here, as I believe that each infant must have the percentage of fat given to it which is adapted to its own peculiar fat digestion; that the successful use of fats depends upon the knowledge of the individual physician of the especial case rather than on invariably using high or low percentages, and that, so far as the nutrition of the infant is concerned, a gradually increasing percentage of fat, according as it can be adapted to the digestion, is indicated, always enunciating that a percentage of fat higher than 4 is only necessary in very unusual cases. So many opinions have been expressed by physicians in regard to the method of obtaining cream for percentage use, and so much prejudice has been shown as regards the use of centrifugal cream, that it may be well to state that gravity cream, as well as centrifugal cream, can always be obtained at the laboratories, and that quite a number of physicians are accustomed in writing their prescriptions to signify their wish that in writing for their percentages of fat, it is to be understood that gravity cream should be used.

There are a number of variations possible and practical in the use of the different carbohydrates, and I have, therefore, thought it worth while to put in prescription form the various carbohydrates, such as lactose (milk sugar), maltose (malt sugar), sucrose (cane sugar), dextrose (grape sugar), and starch. The explanation of many of the successful results in infant

feeding lies in the especial carbohydrate which it is possible to
embody in the various preparations of food. It is now possible
by laboratory methods to prescribe for and obtain any or all of
these carbohydrates which, for so many ·years, have been used
with greater or less success in the patent and proprietary foods.
In order to understand why certain carbohydrates, for instance,
such as maltose, should be rationally used instead of always using
lactose, I would draw your attention to this table (Table I.),
which shows the different kinds of fermentation and the relative rapidity of fermentation which the various sugars undergo,
and I have arranged them in the order of their rapidity of conversion. For instance, in regard to the formation of lactic acid,
lactose is very much more rapid in its conversion into lactic acid
than are dextrose, sucrose and maltose. On the other hand,
where an over amount of butyric acid is interfering with the
digestion, it is well to know that maltose is converted into butyric
acid far more rapidly than are dextrose, sucrose and lactose. As
a result of a knowledge of these facts, we should appreciate that
where there is an excess of lactic acid, maltose should be used
rather than lactose and dextrose, while where butyric acid is over-
produced, lactose is indicated rather than maltose or sucrose.

TABLE I.

* Table I. shows the kinds of fermentation and the relative
rapidity of conversion which the different sugars undergo, arranged in the order of their rapidity :—

LACTIC ACID.	BUTYRIC ACID.	ALCOHOLIC.
Levulose	Levulose	Maltose
Lactose	Maltose	Invert sugar
Dextrose	Dextrose	Sucrose
Invert sugar	Invert sugar	Dextrose
Sucrose	Sucrose	Levulose
Maltose	Lactose	Lactose

Again referring to Table I., the table of the carbohydrates, we
can see how easy it is, having once acquired a knowledge of the
principal ingredients of the patent foods, to simply ignore them

---

* Work done by Altchison Robertson. *Edinburgh Medical Journal,* March, 1894.

as not containing anything of importance beyond what can be provided more precisely and, certainly far cheaper, than when a bottle or can of these foods has to be bought in order to add the important part of any especial patent food to a milk mixture.

For instance, suppose that the physician finds that he has some, as he thinks, unexplained success from the use of a food of which maltose is the principal ingredient. He can then, in place of the lactose, which is so often prescribed in the milk mixtures, use maltose, and he not only is thus giving the infant exactly what has been of benefit to it in the patent food, but also can, by means of careful percentage prescription, determine and give the exact amount of maltose which is suited to the especial infant. The same may be said of preparations where dextrose seems to be indicated, for in this case, physicians have merely to prescribe a certain percentage of dextrose. When the question of another and important member of the carbohydrate group, starch, is to be dealt with, we should consider in what way this especial carbohydrate may be useful in infant feeding. Starch can be used for two purposes: (1) to render the precipitated casein finer by mechanical means, and (2) for purposes of nutrition. We should understand that, for the mechanical virtue of starch, it requires 0.75 per cent. starch to make the precipitate of the casein finer. For purposes of nutrition, each physician must decide for himself how early he considers it well for starch, as a nutrient, to be added to an infant's food, and according as he prefers to call into action the infant's amylolytic function before it has been fully developed, or to wait until such function has been practically developed.

We should also note that when starch is given as a nutrient, the maximum amount which can be prescribed for is represented by 1.30 per cent.

In the technic of dextrinizing starch, we should understand that it requires one hour for complete dextrinization, but that as in intelligently using the other food stuffs we should dextrinize a shorter or longer time, according to the requirements of the especial case.

In connection with this line of thought, I have shown in Table II. the assimilative limit in adults without an overflow of sugar occurring in the urine.

TABLE II.

Possible amount assimilated in twenty-four hours without overflow:—

Lactose	120	grams
Sucrose	150-200	"
Levulose	200	"
Dextrose	200-250	"

In this manner we can, for instance, where for the purpose of nutrition sugars are indicated, use more dextrose than lactose.

I have also shown in Table III. the changes which the carbohydrates undergo before their assimilation in the form of dextrose:—

TABLE III.

Starch is converted into dextrins and then into maltose.
One molecule of maltose is converted into two molecules of dextrose.
One molecule of sucrose is converted into one molecule of dextrose and into one molecule of levulose.
One molecule of lactose is converted into one molecule of dextrose and one of galactose.
Dextrose is the body sugar.

It is well to note also that glycogen, or animal starch, may be formed from dextrose in the liver, where it may be stored, and when needed, changed back into dextrose and then carried from the liver into the general circulation.

If, again, the physician wishes to predigest starch, he can simply signify in his prescription that starch is to be dextrinized, with the understanding that the laboratory will accomplish this with the ferment diastase.

From the above Table III. it will be seen that while the carbohydrates undergo many different changes, one of the final results in each case is dextrose, the only sugar which is capable of being assimilated in the body. Therefore, starch, as a food, undergoes more changes and requires more time for its final conversion than do any of the others. Also, if a carbohydrate be needed for rapid assimilation, dextrose would be the one indicated.

The separation of the principal elements of the proteids in prescribing them in the modification of milk for infant feeding, was a great advance in laboratory possibilities, and has now been accepted by many physicians as a notable addition in the pre-

scribing of milk and in dealing successfully with infantile digestion. It has, in my experience, done away almost entirely with the
necessity of using cereals to make the flocculi of the precipitated ·
casein finer. This question, however, need have nothing to do
with whether the physician is using such cereal for the purpose
of nutrition. This dividing of the proteids accomplishes in much
the most rational way the control of such cases as have difficulty
with the digestion of the casein, and yet need a higher percentage
of the total proteids for nutrition, since in this way of dealing
with the proteids we can give exactly as much casein as is indicated
in the special case, or rather as much as can be readily digested.

The following Table IV. shows the possible combinations
of whey and casein which can be obtained by the milk laboratories
in cases where the fat desired in the prescription is from 1 to 4
per cent. and the sugar from 4 to 7 per cent.

Table IV.

WHEY PROTEIDS. Per Cent.	CASEIN. Per Cent.
0.25	0.25
0.50	0.25
0.75	0.25
0.80	0.25
0.80	0.50
0.80	0.75
0.75	0.50
0.80	0.60
0.80	0.90
0.75	1.15

It should be noted that while in the former prescriptions
emanating from the laboratories the word caseinogen has been
used, casein has now been substituted for it. This change has been
made for the following reason: Casein is a neutral organic com-
pound forming both acid and alkali combinations, while caseinogen simply indicates that it is the mother substance of casein.

While in the past we thought that we were able to obtain .90
per cent. of whey proteids in our prescription, the chemist of the
milk laboratory has now proved that we can be provided with
no higher than .80 per cent.

If, as is sometimes the case, we find that, even with the small
percentage of casein which can be obtained by dividing the proteids, the casein digestion is still weak, we can temporarily obviate

this difficulty by peptonization. In writing our prescription for this purpose, we simply indicate whether peptonization should be carried to such an extent as to render the mixture more or less bitter, or not bitter at all. This is regulated by knowing that twenty minutes gives a decidedly bitter taste.

As so much in recent literature has been said about the introduction of citrate of soda in milk mixtures, it is well to say a few words about this salt before stating exactly what it should be used for, if it is used at all. I have given it a place on the prescription card as, in the minds of certain physicians, it really plays an important rôle.

Citrate of soda is not an alkali, although, so far as its results are concerned, it may take the place of an alkali in connection with the digestion of casein. Citrate of soda, when added to the milk, decalcifies the casein, and as a result the casein is not affected by rennet, and, therefore, forms with the acids of the stomach soft, friable flakes (of the buttermilk type) instead of tough curds.

When sodium citrate is used in place of the alkali, it requires 0.20 per cent. to each ounce of the milk and cream used in modifying to facilitate the digestion of the proteids, and 0.40 per cent. to prevent the action of the rennet, and to ensure the formation in the stomach of soft curds instead of tough ones.

While in health, it is usually not difficult to adapt the percentages of either a divided proteid, or, later, a whole proteid, to the digestive capacity of the infant, yet in certain abnormal conditions, most of us who have had much to do with the gastric disturbances of early life have found a more or less alkaline reaction of the milk mixture to be of aid in our treatment. There are two reasons for producing a greater or less alkalinity in a food mixture: (1) To favor the production of hydrochloric acid in the stomach, and to thus aid in the digestion of the casein. A moderate amount of alkalinity is sufficient for this purpose. (2) If we wish to relieve the stomach from all work in connection with the proteids, we must add sufficient alkali to suspend all action of the stomach on the proteids.

The amount of alkalinity prescribed, or the substances used to produce such alkalinity, should be such as the especial practitioner deems wise for the individual case. As, however, in the majority of the prescriptions which come to the milk laboratories, lime water and bicarbonate of soda are the alkalies asked for,

I shall only mention these two ingredients, and describe what is supposed to be the reason for using them, and how they have been shown to accomplish the best results. If we wish to merely favor or assist the digestion of the proteids, an amount of lime water equal to 20 per cent. of the milk and cream used in the modification of the milk called for should be used. Fifty per cent. of the amount of milk and cream used in the mixture suspends all action of the stomach on the proteids. If the lime water is 5 per cent. of the total mixture, it gives a mildly alkaline food. If bicarbonate of soda is used instead of lime water, it requires 0.68 per cent. of the milk and cream used in modifying the mixture to favor the digestion of the proteids. Bicarbonate of soda 1.7 per cent. of the amount of milk and cream used suspends all action of the stomach on the proteids, and 0.17 per cent. of the total mixture gives a mildly alkaline food.

In connection with what I have said concerning the various carbohydrates which we can now make use of in a food, I have indicated how useless it is to use these patent foods, and it is of some significance to note that most of these foods have acquired their reputation by the use of various ingredients, of which the most common are starch and maltose. The makers of these foods have naturally used the carbohydrates since they are the easiest to deal with on account of their possibilities for entering into a food which will keep for some time when compounded. The notable lack of fats and proteids in the patent foods may be partially explained by the great objection to using these compounds, owing to the difficulty of preserving them.

I am greatly indebted to Mr. Frederic W. Howe, professor of physiological chemistry and dietetics in the State Normal School at Framingham, Mass., both for his explanation of the results of his work on the patent foods and in showing how their use can be done away with. Through Professor Howe I have been enabled to obtain from the laboratory still another addition to our means of facilitating the digestion of the proteids in cases of weak casein digestion, and also for inhibiting the saprophytes of fermentation in disturbances of the intestinal tract, notably in cases of fermental indigestion. This has been accomplished by means of the lactic acid bacillus. The action of this bacillus in reference to facilitating digestion can be stated definitely in the prescription if we recognize what is known of its physiological chemistry. We should know that .25 per cent. of lactic acid just

curdles the milk. .50 per cent. gives a thick curdled milk, while
.75 per cent. separates the milk into curds and whey. Whether
we prescribe one or another of these percentages depends upon
the taste and preference of the individual patient. These percentages represent the per cent. of lactic acid attained when the
food is removed from the thermostat. When the lactic acid
bacillus is used to facilitate the digestion of the proteids, these
percentages represent the final acidity, as the process is then
stopped by heat at this point. When the lactic acid bacillus, on
the contrary, is used to inhibit the growth of saprophytes in
abnormal fermental conditions of the intestines, the acidity may
subsequently increase to a variable degree, as the process is not
stopped at this point since it is desirable for the bacilli to be left
alive.

The practical object of my suggestion to the laboratory authorities to adopt a new prescription blank, was not only to show
the profession how unnecessary it was to encourage the owners
of the patent foods, by buying what can just as well, and cheaper,
be put up at the laboratories, but also to induce the average physician to make use of the more modern methods of treatment.
For this purpose, I have advised explaining on the prescription
blank what we are practically doing when we prescribe for our
patients and how we can become familiar with the more delicate
shades of treatment by using the technique which the laboratories
provide for our convenience and aid.

As a summary, I would say that not only is there no practical
object in making use of the patent foods when we can perfectly
well prescribe whatever is of importance in these foods, but also
that understanding exactly what the food stuffs in a particular
preparation are, and what their physiological and chemical meaning is, we can, by intelligent prescriptions, aid in the development
of a better system of infant feeding.

Although the experience of one individual must only be taken
for what it is worth, it seems to me that many physicians will
agree with me when I say that, in the future, it will be possible
to accomplish in our cases of feeding, both in health and in disease, far more than has ever been done before, and I believe that,
by using this prescription blank which I have brought to your
notice, we shall gain much in the accuracy of our mixtures, in
convenience, in simplicity and in lessening the cost of our mixtures of food.

NEW PRESCRIPTION CARD SUGGESTED BY DR. ROTCH FOR

LABORATORY USE.

Explanatory.		Per cent.
(a) Gravity cream will be used instead of centrifugal, if ordered.	(a) Fats.................................	
(b) The maximum amount of starch possible in any prescription when used as a nutrient is 1.30%. It requires 0.75% starch to make the precipitated casein finer.	(b) Carbohydrates. { Lactose (milk sugar) Maltose (malt sugar) Sucrose (cane sugar) Dextrose (grape sugar) Starch (b)	
(c) One hour completely dextrinizes starch.	(c) Dextrinize..............................	
(d) In case physicians do not wish to subdivide the proteids, the words "Whey" and "Casein" may be erased.	(d) Proteids.........{ Whey......... .... Casein	
(e) It requires 0.20% of the milk and cream used to facilitate the digestion of the proteids, i.e., the formation of a soft curd; 0.40% to prevent the action of rennet, i.e., the formation of a tough curd.	(e) Sodium Citrate...........................	
(f) Twenty minutes renders the mixture decidedly bitter.	(f) Peptonize...............................	
(g) It requires 20% of the milk and cream used in modifying to facilitate the digestion of the proteids. 50% of the amount of milk and cream used suspends all action on the proteids in the stomach. 5% of the total mixture gives a mildly alkaline food.	(g) Lime Water..... { Per cent. of milk and cream.... Per cent. of total mixture	
(h) It requires 0.68% of the milk and cream used in modifying to facilitate the digestion of the proteids. 1.70% of the amount of milk and cream used suspends all action on the proteids in the stomach. 0.17% of the total mixture gives a mildly alkaline food.	(h) Sodium Bicarb.. { Per cent. of milk and cream.... Per cent. of total mixture	
(i) Percentage figures represent the per cent. of lactic acid attained when the food is removed from the thermostat. When the lactic acid bacillus is used to facilitate the digestion of the proteids, the percentage called for represents the final acidity, as the process is stopped by heat at this point. When the lactic acid bacillus is used to inhibit the growth of saprophytes, the acidity may subsequently increase to a variable degree, as the bacilli are left alive. 0.25% lactic acid just curdles milk. 0.50% gives thick curdled milk. 0.75% separates the milk into curds and whey.	(i) Lactic Acid Bacillus { 1. To facilitate digestion of proteids. 2. To inhibit the saprophytes of fermentation.	
	When the lactic acid bacillus is not called for in the prescription, heat at................F... Number of feedings........................ Amount at each feeding ....ounces	

DISCUSSION.

DR. HOLT.—I regret very much that the paper which has been in preparation by Dr. Clarke and myself is not ready to be presented at this meeting and has to be presented by title. A good deal of the work done by Dr. Clarke is along the lines suggested by Dr. Rotch's paper. I will only state one of the experiments—that with lime water. The experiment was made to determine the effect upon the gastric secretion. He used plain milk diluted with water, with lime water, and with soda. The chief effect of the lime water appeared to be an enormous increase in HCl production which took place. (That was very evident when lime water was used.) Gastric digestion goes forward largely according to the amount of HCl present. In no single one of the experiments has there ever been found a deficiency of pepsin in the infant's stomach, but there has been found a great variation in the amount of HCl. The contents of the stomach were removed a half hour after the child was fed and the quantities of different ingredients taken, and these fluids were set aside in a test tube in a thermostat to see what further digestion would take place. He found that in a short time the process came to a rest, but that if more HCl were added it would go on until complete proteid digestion had taken place, showing that the problem was to increase to as great a degree as possible the HCl secretion. The results of these experiments so far indicate that probably the chief advantage of the lime water is that it greatly stimulates the secretion of HCl.

DR. CHAPIN.—It has been a great pleasure to me to hear this paper of Dr. Rotch's, inasmuch as it shows that he recognizes and wishes to apply scientifically the various diluents that many of us have found most useful. As far back as the Deer Park meeting, and later at Niagara, the papers I read on the subject of diluents were written with the same object with which Dr. Rotch has now prepared this paper, namely, recognizing that certain proprietary foods did in many cases do good to find if we could not, as physicians, utilize the good in them in a scientific way. These various food stuffs are valuable, not only from the standpoint of diluents, but from a nutritional standpoint, and that leads me to say that I believe the whole subject of infant feeding can only be satisfactorily discussed from the biological standpoint, not from a chemical standpoint exclusively, and that is the point I have made for quite a number of years. The possibilities and limitations of all plans of infant feeding can only be judged by biology, which means that you must understand the intestinal tract of various animals; that milks are not interchangable in any sense; that milks have a double function, a developmental as well as a nutritive function. The developmental function has been heretofore ignored. That is only one example of how careful biological inductions may help us in this subject of infant feeding.

Dr. Caillé.—Dr. Rotch's method is too complicated and really just as empirical as our simple methods of feeding for this reason: Let us assume that we have three test tubes and in one we place water and nitrate of silver and chloride of sodium in certain proportions. The chemist will be able to tell us the qualitative and quantitative end results. Now take the gastroenteric tract as another test tube; you place in a definite quantity of your food, your milk, fats, proteids, sugars and salts, but the secretions and bacteria are not always the same, and the motor efficiency of the digestive tract varies. There is no one who can tell us the end results under such conditions. Now, assume the gastroenteric tract to be invaded by pathogenic bacteria or infected, where is the brain that will tell us the end results? That is my difficulty in attempting to teach others a method of feeding which can be managed only in the hands of a few persons and which is at best empirical. I admire the scientific study of feeding, but I teach the practitioner practical methods.

Dr. Griffith.—I am a thorough believer in the principles and practice of percentage feeding, and I work on no other plan. At the same time it seems to me that every effort should be made to keep the matter *evidently,* as well as really, simple, if we expect the profession in general to follow it. The new formula-blanks, which Dr. Rotch presents, look a little complicated, although really not so.

Dr. Northrup.—One of the ingredients has scarcely been mentioned and that is the milk. I think it would be well to put into these feedings milk. One of the great triumphs of the laboratory, to my mind, has been that they have given us an object lesson in the production of a pure milk with a known fat content of unvarying degree.

Dr. Rotch.—I have always felt very grateful to the members of this Society for the way in which they have thoroughly discussed this subject. It shows that they are all interested in it, and that we are all working in the same direction. It speaks well for a subject that it provokes discussion. But we are a little inclined, I think, to wander away from the real principle. Of course, we know that the milk supply is the keynote to the whole situation and that we are trying to improve it all the time. The great improvement that has already been made is wonderful.

Remember that we are trying to learn which are the best instruments to work with, just as you would do with surgical instruments. I am simply taking up what I think is an advance in infant feeding, namely, why it is that some foods agree with babies better than others. Is it not an advance to learn why one of these is better than another? As to the alkalinity, I am not an exponent as an individual, but I am making use of our combined knowledge on the subject. Dr. Southworth, for instance, has given us the most advanced teaching as to alkalinity.

Again, Dr. Dunn can show case after case where this lactic acid feeding has not been unavailing. These cases have done better than any set of cases that we have previously treated.

Dr. Caillé says only a few persons know how to use percentage feeding; he is mistaken. There are many men who know how to use it and are doing so. No one should attempt to throw cold water upon these investigations. I do not ignore in any way the great possibilities of human milk. We are beginning to understand more and more why it is better than any modified milk, when it is good, but we cannot get it over and over again, and we should endeavor, when we cannot get good human milk, to get the best modification we can.

Dr. Jacobi.—I do not understand the difference that has been claimed between chemistry and biology. I do not see that there is any boundary line between the two. If there were we should not be in a position to speak of and study biological chemistry. We should not have the very efficient and learned journal coming regularly on the subject of biological chemistry. I do not recognize that boundary line, and therefore I think Dr. Chapin is not justified from that point of view in bringing up that issue. I believe that Dr. Rotch and Dr. Chapin work on the same basis. It is an increase in our knowledge of organic chemistry that we do not make this distinction any more. Biology cannot exist without chemistry; and biochemistry will become the biology of the future more and more.

Dr. Chapin.—I did not intend to put biology against chemistry, but to protest against putting a chemical value on foods to the exclusion of their biologic value.

Dr. Jacobi.—We should not forget that we cannot all work in the same line. There is not a man in the profession in America that has done more original work on just these points, the study of the chemistry and biology of milk, than our friend Dr. Rotch. There are two classes of men among us: those who do original work and those who have more critical minds. We have here a few who do original work; the majority of us, myself included, have only the critical mind. Let us be satisfied that both of these classes, and all of us here who belong to one or the other, have the same purpose in view.

THE HARD CURDS OF INFANT STOOLS; THEIR ORIGIN, NATURE AND TRANSFORMATION.

BY THOMAS S. SOUTHWORTH, M.D.,

AND

OSCAR M. SCHLOSS, M.D.,
New York.

The discovery that the firm rounded curds, occurring not infrequently in the stools of infants fed upon cow's milk, are composed in part of fatty acids and soaps has led to considerable discussion and seems to warrant a further inquiry into the origin of such bodies and their subsequent transformation during their passage through the digestive tract. The claim has frequently been made of late that these masses are simply aggregations of soaps and fatty acids containing no proteid and therefore by implication are not entitled to be called curds. Although doubtless founded upon some individual tests, this view of the hard curd seems to be largely based upon the categorical statement of Czerny and Keller* in discussing "casein stools" that "these flakes and masses which have been taken for casein in the feces are not casein, but fatty soaps."

It is not an uncommon experience to find in the vomited matter both of sick adults and of infants with disturbed digestions, when upon a milk diet, large firm rounded and somewhat elongated masses of rubbery consistency which are assumed to be the result of the coagulation of cow's milk under abnormal stomachic conditions. It is at least inconceivable that these vomited masses have been formed anywhere else than in the stomach, and they correspond, moreover, very closely in appearance to the curds which may be formed from cow's milk by the addition of rennet-pepsin and acid, heating the mixture to body temperature and, when the whole has coagulated, pressing the coagulum repeatedly together so as to thoroughly expel the whey. Such masses formed artificially no one certainly hesitates to call a curd, for when thus formed experimentally outside the body by the process above outlined the product differs in no essential particular from the early stages of the curd of ordinary commercial cheddar cheese. The conditions which are necessary for the formation of a cheesy milk

---

* Des Kindes Ernährung, Erhährungsstörungen und Ernährungstheraple, s. 17; Sechste abteilung, zweite hälfte, 1906.

curd, namely, rennet-pepsin, acid, warmth and pressure, may also be present in an infant's stomach, especially during those types of disturbed digestion which increase the amount of abnormal acids. The only real difference then between the factors in the commercial and physiological production of curds lies in the fact that while lactic acid is chiefly active in the commercial process, hydrochloric, butyric, acetic and other acids may also play a part in the stomach.

The curds formed from milk, although often spoken of as acid-paracasein curds, or loosely as "casein curds," because of the major part necessarily played in their formation by the coagulation and curding of casein, are not, however, composed exclusively of paracasein. In the formation of a cheese curd the fat of the milk is included in the meshes of the paracasein coagulum, and only a small part of this fat (less than 0.50 per cent.) escapes in the whey.

To understand the subsequent changes in these curds if formed in the stomach of the infant, it is therefore important to keep in mind that they are milk curds, including both fat and paracasein. If curding has taken place in small flakes these can be more or less thoroughly penetrated and affected by the proteolytic and fat-splitting ferments present in the stomach. But if large and compact these masses frequently cannot be disintegrated in the stomach, although it is possible that both fat and proteid may undergo some changes more especially upon the exposed surface. When not disintegrated in the stomach these masses, unless vomited, must in time be passed on into the intestines, where they are subjected to the further influences of an alkaline medium, the fat-splitting and saponifying agencies of the hepatic, pancreatic and intestinal secretions, and the destructive action of the varied bacterial flora there present. In the intestine, fats are split by ferments into glycerin and fatty acids, and the latter, in an alkaline medium, may be more or less transformed into soluble or insoluble soaps according to the nature of the bases with which they combine. When the proteid network is accessible it is subjected to digestive action, and bacteria which flourish upon proteid material may penetrate to some extent into its structure. Small soft flakes, if intestinal conditions are normal, may thus be readily disintegrated, while the larger masses may not be disintegrated, and may eventually appear in the stools.

Howland has recently advanced the view that the occurrence of such masses in the stools is an evidence of excessive fat in the infant's food. The formation of such curds in the stomach is not limited to cases receiving a high percentage of fat in their food, since observation directed to this point will show that they occur even with very considerable dilutions of plain milk, and the explanation of their occurrence in Howland's type of cases need not be a difficult one. Since high fat percentages frequently cause stomachic disturbances, accompanied by the production of excessive quantities of abnormal acids, the most favorable condition is present for the formation of large curds, namely, excessive acidity. Furthermore, the larger the amount of fat in the milk food, the larger the fat inclusion in the proteid coagulum, the larger the mass formed, and the less the probability that it can be disintegrated during its passage through the digestive tract, since the greater preponderance of fat will tend to weld it the more firmly together.

If further argument is needed to prove that the formation of these masses depends primarily upon the coagulation and curding of the paracasein, it may be found in the effect of efficient peptonization. Peptonization of milk which transforms such portions of the casein as its action reaches into soluble and non-coagulable forms of proteid is one of the best recognized of available methods for causing the disappearance of such masses from the stools. It should be remembered, however, that this result is not always attained because the partial peptonization so often employed may leave considerable casein unaltered and still capable of entering into the formation of large curds. Citrate of soda, lauded for this purpose by Wright, and certain alkalies may also be effective, the former by preventing the formation of paracasein and the latter by delaying curding and by neutralizing excessive and abnormal acidity. However, all these must be used in sufficient quantity.

Although the foregoing theoretical and clinical grounds for considering the masses found in the stools to be identical in origin with those found in vomited matter seemed reasonably conclusive, a series of observations and tests were instituted at the Nursery and Child's Hospital to definitely settle certain disputed points. Foremost among these was the claim that the masses in the stools contain no proteid, but only fatty acids and soaps.

Typical firm curds occurring in seventy-five stools passed by thirty-eight infants were subjected to qualitative chemical tests to determine the presence of proteids, soaps, fatty acids and neutral fat in these masses. In the tabulation of the results the tests upon the stools of older children who were receiving whole milk together with other diet consisting of eggs, cereals, etc., have, with the exception of two representative instances (numbers 25 and 26), been excluded in the belief that the findings among younger infants fed exclusively upon milk formulas would prove of greater interest. In the table as appended appear the tests upon masses found in fifty-one stools of twenty-six infants. The youngest were two months old. Ten were from two to six months old. Eleven from seven to thirteen months old. One fifteen months old and two three years old. The fat in the formulas varied from 2 per cent. to 4 per cent. In only five cases did it exceed 3 per cent. The proteid percentages ranged from 0.90 per cent. to 4 per cent. In but eight of these, however, did the proteid exceed 2.50 per cent., and the majority of these were older infants fed upon plain milk diluted with barley gruel. Few, if any, of the formulas seem open to criticism as excessive if fed to normal infants at the ages given.

The technique employed was as follows:—

(1) The masses to be tested were ground in a mortar and thoroughly treated with successive portions of ether and boiling alcohol to dissolve out the neutral fat and free fatty acids. These solvents were then evaporated and their residue examined microscopically for fatty acid crystals (often after recrystallizing from boiling alcohol) and also tested with osmic acid and Sudan III. for fat.

(2) The residue remaining after ether and alcohol extraction was then treated with 5 per cent. hydrochloric acid which would split the insoluble soaps into fatty acids and form chlorides of the bases, as well as remove any inorganic salts. The residue was then again treated thoroughly with boiling alcohol to remove any fatty acid thus formed and the remainder washed with ether, thoroughly dried and set aside for the proteid tests. The washings (alcoholic) were examined for fatty acids, the finding of which at this stage would indicate the presence of insoluble soaps in the original masses.

(3) The washed and dried residue was then in each instance

subjected to each of four well-known tests for proteids. These were the Biuret, Lieberman's, Millon's and Adamkiewicz's tests.

Applying these qualitative methods to the firm masses or hard curds, these bodies were found to consist mainly of fatty acids and protein in varying amounts, although they showed uniformly the presence of neutral fat by the staining reactions. Insoluble soaps were often present but apparently in lesser amounts than is usually assumed, never appearing in these purely qualitative tests to approach in amount the fatty acid or the protein. In some of the curds the final residue considered to be protein was at least one-half of the original mass tested. In every instance without exception, the final residue of the masses responded to all four of the tests for protein. Bearing in mind that a possible source of error might lie in the presence of bacteria which might give the protein reactions, the masses were in thirty instances examined for bacteria by staining smears with aniline gentian violet, and in no instance were they found to be numerous. As a further and more important control the stool substance in which the masses were found was in every case subjected to exactly the same processes and tests and in no instance could the presence of protein be demonstrated. In order to ascertain whether soluble soaps were present in these masses and had been dissolved out by the first treatment with ether and boiling alcohol eleven hard curds from the stools of nine infants were examined for soluble soaps and in no case were they found.

The characteristic masses upon which this series of tests were made varied usually in size from that of a small pea to that of the last phalanx of the adult thumb. Their surface was usually smooth and their shape rounded or oval. In some cases they showed irregularities and indentations due to pressure against each other. They were often quite hard so that it took considerable force to cut them. At other times they were so soft that they could be smoothed out with very little pressure. The hardness depended upon the relative amount of proteid, soaps, fatty acids and neutral fat present. The softer ones consisted mainly of fatty acid or fat, while the harder masses contained a relatively greater amount of protein. In the typical hard curd the cut surface showed a structure resembling closely that of curds made artificially or of those vomited by infants. The masses containing considerable fatty acid were white, translucent, very soft and friable and easily obliterated by pressure, while those which contained protein chiefly were hard, opaque, of a yellowish white color upon the surface and could not be obliterated by moderate pressure. The masses rich in fat and fatty acids were often flattened and partially melted when seen in the fresh stool. These softer masses consisting largely of fatty acids and fat melted almost completely with moderate heat, while the masses richer in protein melted less completely and on increasing the heat had the appearance and odor of toasted cheese.

We would repeat that all of these masses responded to the tests for proteids no matter whether they were hard or soft and regardless of the presence of soaps, neutral fat or fatty acid. On the other hand the ordinary stool substance in which these masses were imbedded when subjected to the same procedure and tests did not give the protein reactions.

There are, however, certain other masses occurring in the stools of infants both those who are nursed, and those who are artificially fed which are made up practically of calcium soaps alone, but these masses can hardly be mistaken for true curds. They are quite small, rarely larger than .2 to .3 c.m. in diameter. They usually occur in green or greenish stools from which they are distinguishable by their gray color. They are very soft, can be flattened out by pressure, are not friable, and are a more homogeneous part of the stool mass than the true curd.

Two of the cases tabulated (Numbers 9 and 8) are of especial interest as bearing upon the origin of true curds. The first (Case 9) an infant of six months and weighing thirteen pounds, had been receiving without disturbance a split proteid formula: Fat, 3 per cent.; sugar, 6 per cent.; whey proteid, 0.90 per cent.; casein, 1.10 per cent., which was changed to an ordinary F 3.—S 6.—P 2. formula. Vomiting of curds ensued and hard rounded masses appeared in the stools consisting largely of protein. On resuming the split proteid formula the vomiting and the curds in the stools disappeared. The second case (Case 8) was almost identical, a change being made from: Fat, 3 per cent.; sugar, 6 per cent.; whey proteid, 0.90; casein, 0.70 per cent. to an ordinary F 3.—S 6.—P. 1.60 formula. In this case also vomiting and curds ceased on resuming the previous formula.

It therefore seems apparent that the observation of others that

TABLE OF MATERIAL TESTED.

Name.	Age.	Formula.	Reaction of Stool with Litmus.	Protein.	Fatty Acid.	Neutral Fat.	Soaps.
1. D. F.	2 mos.	3 —6—1	acid	+	++	+	+
2. M. L.	2 "	2.50—6—1	"	++	++	+	+
3. A. W.	3 "	2.50—5—1	"	+++	+	+	+
4. E. H.	3½"	3 —6—1.50	"	+++	+	+	+
"	" "	"	"	+++	+	+	+
"	"	"	"	+++	+		
5. J. S.	4 "	2 —6—1.50	"	+	+	++	
6. J. K.	5 "	2.50—5—1.50	"	+	++	+	—?
7. A. L.	6 "	2 —6—2 B.W.	"	++	+	+	+?
8. C. O.	6 "	2.50—6—1.60	"	+	+	+	—?
9. J. E.	6 "	3 —6—2	"	++	+	+	+
"	" "	"	"	++	+	+	+
10. J. A.	6 "	3 —6—2	"	++	++	+	+
11. A. L.	7 "	2.50—6—2	"	++	+	+	+
12. T. K.	7 "	2 —6—.90	"	+	+	++	+
"	" "	"	"	+	+	++	+
13. J. S.	7 "	2.50—7—2	"	++	+	+	+
"	" "	"	"	++	+	+	—?
14. A. S.	8 "	2 —6—2 B.W.	"	++	++	+	+
15. H. H.	8 "	3 —6—3 B.W.	"	++	++	+	—?
"	" "	"	"	++	++	+	—?
16. M. H.	8 "	3 —6 { .90 whey proteid / 1.10 casein }	"	+++	+	+	+
"	" "	"	"	+	++	+	—?
"	" "	"	"	+	++	+	+
17. W. R.	8 "	4 —7—3	"	++	++	+	+?
"	" "	"	"	++	++	+	
18. A. T.	1 yr.	3 —6—3 B.W.	"	+++	+	+	+
"	" "	"	"	+	+++	+	—?
"	" "	"	"	+	+	+	+
"	" "	"	"	+	+	+	++
19. J. A.	1 "	3.50—6—3.50 B.W.	"	+	+	+	+
20. M. C.	1 "	3.50—6—2.50	"	++	+	+	+
"	" "	"	"	+	+	+	+
21. O. L.	1 "	2 —6—2 B.W.	"	+	++	+	+
"	" "	"	"	+	++	+	+
22. P. P.	1 "	3 —6—3 B.W.	"	++	+	+	+
"	" "	"	alkaline	+	+++	+	—?
"	" "	"	acid	++	++	+	+
23. J. M.	13 mos.	3 —6—3 B.W.	"	+++	+++	+	+
"	" "	"	"	+	+++	+	+
"	" "	"	"	+	+++	+	—?
24. J. W.	15 "	3 —4—3 B.W.	"	+++	+	+	+
25. B. F.	3 yrs.	whole milk, cereal, eggs, etc.	alka.	+	+++	+	+
"	" "	"	acid	++	++	+	+
26. I. T.	3 "	whole milk, cereal, eggs, etc.	"	+++	+	+	+
"	" "	"	"	+	+++	+	+
"	" "	"	"	+	+++	+	+

In the above table the plus signs are to be interpreted as follows:—

+ slight amount.   B. W. = Barley Water.

++ moderate amount.

+++ large amount.

these typical masses contained considerable fatty acid, neutral fat and soaps has led to the hasty conclusion that the masses were simply aggregations of fat derivatives and not true curds. No confusion need, however, arise on this score if we draw upon our available knowledge concerning the curding of milk in the stomach and recall that by all analogies as well as by chemical tests of such curds whether when rejected from the stomach by vomiting or passed on through the intestine, such firm massive curds must primarily be "milk curds" whose origin depends upon the formation of acid paracasein and that the inclusion of fat is but an inevitable mechanical accident.

DISCUSSION.

ISAAC A. ABT, M.D., Chicago.—There is no more fertile field for investigation than the subject under discussion, particularly in view of the investigations made abroad. The results that have been reported from the Berlin school and the Breslau school, would lead us to believe that there is no such thing as proteid indigestion. The statement made by Czerny and Keller, in their most excellent treatise, goes on to say that if the chapter on the subject of digestion of food had been written ten years before they would have said that all disturbances were due to proteid indigestion, but now they feel that the trouble is entirely due to fats. They also say that the curds in the stool are not formed of proteid, but are a combination of fatty acids and alkalies to form soaps. I have fed babies that suffered from what I presumed was fat indigestion on absolutely fat-free milk and found in stools a curd that corresponds to the one Dr. Southworth has described. It is difficult to understand how a fat-free milk could produce a fat indigestion. I believe this line of investigation is of great importance.

JOHN LOVETT MORSE, M.D., Boston.—My assistant, Dr. Talbot, has been at work on this same subject and has gone into it even more elaborately than Dr. Southworth and his assistant, in that he has worked the thing out quantitatively as well as qualitatively. He has found that the basis of these large curds is in every case a proteid. He has also found that the amount of fat which is present in the curd varies almost exactly with the amount of fat in the food, showing that the fat is merely caught in the meshes of the curd. He has not only found this to be the fact in the curds in babies' stools, but has also found, as would be expected, that the same rule holds good in the artificial digestion of milks containing a varying amount of fat, viz., that the amount of fat in the curd varies with the amount of fat in the milk. His results as to the form of the fat, if I am not mistaken, are different from the results of Dr. Southworth. In the large curds the greater part of the fat was in the form of neutral fat. He has gone a little way into the investigation of the small curds; that is, those about the size of a shot, and has found so far that these curds are composed largely of soaps. The reaction of the stools, if I am not mistaken, depends upon the relation of the fat and proteid in the original food rather than on anything else. We had the same experience that Dr. Southworth did—that we sometimes got these large curds in babies that were taking barley-water mixtures.

S. McC. HAMILL, M.D., Philadelphia.—One year ago I had under my care Dr. Edsall's baby. He was suffering from a mild intestinal disturbance. We added a dextrinized gruel to his milk and within about three days the child began to pass curds which had very much the appearance of those which Dr. Southworth has described.

To determine what relationship the gruel might bear to the curd formation, Dr. Edsall undertook some laboratory experiments with the dextrinized foods. He applied varying amounts of HCl; first, to milk mixtures, and then to milk mixtures containing the gruel. The curd from the milk alone could be readily broken up, but that which resulted from the milk and gruel mixture was a gluey, indestructible mass. These results were so suggestive that we immediately cut out the dextrinized gruels and the curds promptly disappeared, from which we assumed that the laboratory experiment had been confirmed. We further assumed that there was some disturbance of the secreting property of the stomach. There are evidently conditions in which the gruels defeat the purpose for which they are administered, a fact which may throw some light upon this question of curd formation.

DR. NORTHRUP.—I should like to ask Dr. Hamill if the feedings were 5 per cent. alkaline?

DR. HAMILL.—Yes.

CHARLES G. KERLEY, M.D., New York.—Personally, I have used gruels in feeding for a long while, but by their use I have never been able in any one of these cases of proteid incapacity to give a higher percentage. I used them because of the additional nutrition furnished patients, but have not found that a higher proteid percentage could be given because of the introduction of the gruel into the food.

THOMAS S. SOUTHWORTH, M.D., New York (closing discussion).—I appreciate what Dr. Abt has said. I think it is largely due to the writings of Czerny and Keller that there has been this doubt as to the composition of the curd. It seems to me that it has been possible to disprove what the Germans have said, and I am glad to hear Dr. Morse say his own investigations have substantiated ours.

FRESH AIR IN THE TREATMENT OF DISEASE.

BY W. P. NORTHRUP, M.D.,
New York.

There are two points to be discussed: First, the class of cases to which this treatment is especially adapted and in which it has been thoroughly tried; second, the practical application of the method, its working out in detail after much observation and experience.

There is no doubt that open-air, boldly administered, is a method of cure; that it is being promptly accepted and almost universally adopted by the younger members of the profession, and that it has come to stay.

The title reads "fresh air," etc. I could wish that it had in some way included the words "open air," "cool air," or "cold, flowing air." Every musty text-book in the back row of the stack-room ceremoniously includes under "treatment" the words "fresh air," and forthwith proceeds to recommend exclusion of drafts, to hint at blankets in the windows, lint in the sash cracks, etc. In other words, "fresh air" is an indefinite term, a conventional expression, and may mean nothing.

Hot air may contain the requisite oxygen, cellar air may be cool, both may miss the invigorating effect so conspicuously present in open air; that is, in uninclosed, atmospheric air. If it ever is entered in the U. S. P. and standardized for therapeutic use, it should read something like this: "Open air, or cold, fresh, flowing out-door air, dosage regulated to individual needs."

SOME OF THE PHYSIOLOGICAL EFFECTS OF COLD, OPEN AIR.

When the New York Health Department first began to put the tuberculous insane out in the open air to sleep, in shacks, the first important observation noted was, that the patients *slept*, slept without their usual sleeping mixture, *without dope.* This was the regular result. I have observed the same in fever children. From being restless, dusky, and even delirious, they become quiet, of good color and given over to sleep. They often sleep for several hours together, quietly. Next, it is noted that they take their food better; finally that recovery is hastened and completed earlier. These remarks apply more completely to those acutely sick, dopy from toxemia, their case running an acute course. Pneumonia furnishes the best illustration of an acute infectious disease benefited by open-air treatment.

CLASS OF CASES.

I am most familiar with the open-air treatment of pneumonia, scarlet fever and several of the exanthemata, including those with bronchitis and marked cough. I do not hesitate in any of the above cases to put them out of doors in all sorts of weather. As to measles, I am not prepared to state that I have had much experience. I leave it to the members of this society to say whether measles, with its accompanying moist skin, its bronchitis, its tendency to ear complications and its lurking tendencies to accidents, shall be put out of doors. To be consistent, I should say these accidents are due to spreading infectious lesions, and that out-door air would not unfavorably affect them, but at this moment, I am not willing to give a final judgment. I may add just here, that apart from measles, I do not hesitate to put in the open air bronchitis, nasopharyngitis and laryngitis. I do not find that the cough is made worse or the lesions increased. Rather the contrary; the cough becomes less and sleep follows.

PRACTICAL APPLICATION.

In speaking of open-air treatment, I have constantly in mind the conveniences and methods to be observed at the Presbyterian Hospital (New York), open-air ward. A cold ward, or cold open room, presupposes an adjacent warm "grooming" room. Dressing and washing of patients should be done in warm rooms. Patients when once made comfortable, can then be exposed for hours to cool or cold fresh flowing air, and remain comfortable. Here let me say—*the patients and nurses should be made comfortable all the time.* The nurses should wear overcoats or blankets about their shoulders. They have not the appearance of thoroughly applying the open-air treatment in winter until they wear heavy wraps. The patients should be comfortable; then they will like the treatment. To this end the dressing of the bed should be carefully studied out. The following is our present plan in the Presbyterian Hospital. The first requisite is that there should be as much bedding below the patient as above. First a huge, enveloping, extra-sized blanket should be spread upon the bedsprings. Upon this, a rubber blanket or thick paper; then the mattress; upon this a blanket; upon this, again, the sheets, and over these other blankets. After the patient has been well tucked in with the usual bed-blankets, the aforesaid extra-sized, first blanket should be brought round the sides and up from the foot and pinned from chin to toe. At last, the top surface of the bed should look like a huge postal envelope fastened along the middle line, the foot piece coming up to be joined to that line. The copious head folds should envelop the mattress and come down beside the head, the face and chin just emerging. The primal requisition is to construct a huge bag in which the patient may move somewhat without air getting in between the blankets. One other requisite is that the patient should wear a complete suit of light flannel underwear under the nightdress. Whether he wear a night-cap may depend on the individual patient's wishes, upon the amount of hair, etc., etc. He *must* be made comfortable.

In presenting the subject for discussion, these two points have been emphasized:

(1) All febrile cases, measles possibly excepted, may be safely and to advantage treated in the open air.

(2) The comfort of patient and nurses is essential.

To this end the bed must be carefully prepared, as much clothing below the patient as above. The patient should wear a complete flannel suit next to the skin. The nurses should have no false pride about wrapping themselves sufficiently to be comfortable. The best success is to be obtained only in facing the problem fairly and taking for a motto: "Make everyone comfortable."

RESULT.

I have no percentages, no tabulations to present. The success of the treatment must rest on the individual impressions of those making use of it. My own impressions and convictions from my own experience justify the following statement: *Open-air treatment has killed no one, has injured no one, has helped everyone, and determined a cure in a few.*

FRESH AIR IN THE TREATMENT OF DISEASE.

BY EDWIN E. GRAHAM, M.D.,

Professor of Diseases of Children in The Jefferson Medical College, Philadelphia.

One must always study all the factors leading up to, and possibly causing disease, and before deciding the positive influence of one factor, eliminate wholly or in part, other etiological influences.

In considering, therefore, the rôle that fresh air plays, "controls" should be employed, as far as possible, for the comparison of a series of cases of the same disease in the same type of cases living under similar conditions, should enable one to draw fairly accurate conclusions.

My first work in fresh air treatment began some eight years ago in the children's ward of the Philadelphia Hospital. The wards were large, the milk fairly good, enough nurses were on duty to keep the children fed according to my directions, they were bathed regularly and kept clean; but in the wards where the very young infants, mostly foundlings, were placed, the results were very unsatisfactory. Much depended upon the physical condition of the infant on admission. A frail infant, perhaps premature and under normal weight, would gain for a few weeks at best, then remain stationary in weight, finally gradually lose weight, begin to have diarrhea and die. Robust infants on admission often did well for three months. The same symptoms after this period began to develop as in the infants admitted in a condition of malnutrition and in spite of my best efforts, many of these robust children died.

The same type of infants in my private practice were almost without exception, doing well. Convinced that neither the food, nursing, nor general care of these hospital infants was at fault, and that the so-called hospitalism was nothing but lack of fresh air, and lack of out-door air, I ordered these children, in the month of January, placed for two hours each day on the fire-escapes.

The cribs were simply moved out upon the fire-escapes, and

towels pinned over the top of both ends of the crib, as wind shields. The infant mortality began to lessen immediately, and I began to see some hope for my infant hospital patients. In the following two or three years, during my service in January, February and March of each year, I had the children, for a number of hours each day, unless it was raining or snowing, carried down to the large open space facing the hospital buildings, and kept in small hammocks. These infants were always bundled up in blankets, their heads well covered, and their eyes, nose and mouth covered with a gauze veil. They did remarkably well; so well, in fact, that instead of my infants dying, most of them began to gain in weight and health, and the deaths were almost entirely in infants under three months of age, whose condition was distinctly bad upon admission to the hospital.

During the past five years the infants have been placed in the new modern and up-to-date building of the Philadelphia Hospital. The wards are large, the air space ample, the milk the very best; porches surround the hospital on two sides, the infants practically have an abundance of fresh air day and night, and they do as well as could be hoped for. I am no longer a pessimist when in the infants' ward, but an optimist. In the new Jefferson Hospital, where I am on duty the entire year, the children have an ideal ward on the eighth floor, large windows on three sides with a large roof garden adjoining, the latter fitted up with every convenience, such as hammocks, shade, wind shields, etc. The roof garden is used all the year round, winter and summer, and the results are most encouraging.

Of all the factors which have contributed to the reduction of this infant mortality, fresh air has, in my opinion, been the one of prime importance.

During the last three years in my service in the Philadelphia Hospital, I have treated all my severe cases of broncho and lobar pneumonia in children of all ages by the fresh air treatment. These infants and children, as soon as taken ill, are removed from the general ward and placed in a special room provided for such cases. The room holds six cribs comfortably, and rarely, during my service in the last three years, has a bed been vacant. Many of these cases are secondary bronchopneumonia. A large percentage of the children, in fact most of them, are hospital children, but the results have been so different from the old plan as followed years ago, that I have lost more or less my dread of pneumonia as a hospital disease. True, these cases have good nursing, good care and every possible attention, but still they are cases of pneumonia in hospital practice and they do remarkably well.

In another similar room in the same hospital, during the same period of time, I have been treating my typhoids. Occasionally, I have a typhoid under two years of age, most of them are over three, and the average age about six years. The typhoid cases come from the same class of patients as the pneumonias, and they do so much better in the fresh air that nothing could persuade me to return to the old method of treatment, similar in every way to the present, but *minus* the fresh air. The rooms where the typhoids and pneumonias are kept have large windows on two sides, and an open door on a third side; these are kept open day and night; a distinct effort is made to keep the hands and feet of these children warm by gloves, stockings and hot-water bags, but the rooms are always cold, except for a few minutes every two or three hours, when the windows are closed and all the children carefully examined as to cleanliness, etc.

The few cases of tuberculosis are kept in a special portion of one of the porches, living practically in the open air. Arrangements are just being made for a special pavilion for these cases. In the Jefferson Hospital the pneumonia and typhoid cases are treated by the fresh air method and do infinitely better than formerly, when the fresh air treatment was not employed.

In private practice for five years I have treated all infants and children, sick and well, with fresh air; in fact, on my first visit to the child, I, if possible, instill into the mother the principle that fresh air differs from impure air as much as fresh milk from impure milk. Once gain her consent, and the treatment is an assured fact. I am more than surprised to see the willingness with which most mothers, no matter what their social status may be, enter into the treatment. The physician must be enthusiastic; the mother is, in my experience, easy to convince. It would be easy for me to give the histories of cases, but the time allotted to me is brief. Suffice it to say, that in many cases during the winters and summers of the past five years, I have kept numerous infants out of doors all day long, except bringing them in occasionally to the house for the purpose of removing soiled clothing, and I have never in all that time seen a single injurious symptom result, and I am positive it has been the means of saving many lives. Rickets, scrofulosis, gastrointestinal disease, any and all conditions are benefited by the treatment. Measles, in hospital cases, I treat in separate rooms, each room opening upon a common porch, surrounded by glass. During the first few days the children are kept in the cool, darkened rooms, then moved to cribs on the porch, and the windows on the porch opened more or less, insuring an abundance of fresh air. The influence of climate associated with rest in the treatment of nephritis and cardiac disease is now so well recognized that comment is unnecessary.

It is an interesting question, which experience alone can decide, as to what arrangement will, in the future, be made to control the *degree* of temperature in which these children are kept when in the fresh air. In hospital practice it has been my custom to keep infants under three months for a few days in the cool air of the ward before putting them outdoors—the temperature of the ward usually being near 60°F. in the cooler months. In private practice, where the temperature can be more absolutely controlled for each individual case, I gradually but rapidly lower the temperature of the room to 60°F., then dressing the child exactly as if it were to be taken outdoors, gradually lower the temperature of the room for a few hours each day until it approximates the degree of temperature in the fresh outside air. Indifferent temperature feels neither warm nor cold (Wachenheim), and is most restful. In children, indifferent temperature is above 75°F. in summer in summer clothing, and above 65°F. in winter in winter clothing, and varies with age and vitality. Temperatures above indifferent are not sedative, but cause a continuous stimulation that is harmful if prolonged, ending in exhaustion. The same author says that, "Young children stand severe cold badly." This is not my experience, if by "severe cold" is meant the ordinary winter weather in Philadelphia. True it is, that these children are bundled up from head to foot, lie in a comfortable baby coach, and have thick gloves, stockings, veil and perhaps a hot-water bag, but they do breathe the cool air, and they all do well. Two or three rainy or snowy days will convince any one; the children are kept indoors in a warm room and they fuss and cry; out of doors they are quiet.

Humidity has an influence by checking or increasing the evaporation from the body and further studies along this line will be of value.

The distance above sea level exerts a certain distinct influence upon the skin, kidneys and blood, and induces metabolic changes of importance. The influence of a few months of camp life on growing boys is appreciated by every one. "Camp life" is fresh air treatment.

When it is possible to select the kind of fresh air desired, certain broad lines may be followed. Increase of heat production, and, consequently, an augmented metabolism, are rendered necessary by cold, dry air of high altitudes. This is proven by the larger amount of carbonic acid gas given off by the lungs. It also, as a rule, increases the red blood cells during the first few weeks of treatment. High altitudes are useful in children with incipient tuberculosis, or an inherited tendency to tuberculosis.

Fresh seashore air is of decided benefit in infants and children convalescing from severe illnesses, especially gastrointestinal in type. It is of distinct benefit in the so-called strumous type.

Fresh country air is better than fresh city air. Rural districts are better than urban, but density of population, such as one sees often in large cities, does not necessarily imply lack of fresh air. The number of people living in a given area may be very large, but if they live in comfortable houses, keep the windows open and live under the best hygienic conditions, fresh air can be secured in abundance, and infants and children do well. If the same number of people living in the same area do not have an abundance of fresh air, the infants and children do badly. Density of population may have much or little to do with fresh air.

Statistics prove conclusively that in *all* countries where the mothers work in industrial plants, necessitating their absence from home a large portion of the day, that the infants and children show a much higher mortality rate, owing to the fact of their being kept indoors, than among the children of the same class of people living under exactly similar conditions *except* that the mothers live at home and have time to keep their children in the fresh air.

In Berlin, 1903, Newman investigated 2,701 infant deaths. Where the families were in one-room dwellings he found 1,792 deaths; in two-room dwellings, 754 deaths; in three-room dwellings, 122 deaths; in larger dwellings, 43 deaths. Can anything prove more conclusively than this, the power fresh air has to preserve life, or the rapidity with which bad or impure air can cause death? Unfortunately for the infant and young child, the ignorance of many mothers, the superstitions and traditions of others, and the carelessness of a few, are the greatest barriers to the keeping the children in the fresh air. During the past few years comparatively little has been written upon the importance of fresh air for very young children, and yet the subject of fresh air as an aid in the treatment of disease is not of recent date. In the History of the Medical Society of the State of New York, as published in the *New York State Journal of Medicine*, it is shown that in the early part of the nineteenth century the dangers of dust laden air were recognized; the influence that certain occupations exerted upon the etiology of tuberculosis was appreciated, and even at that date "cold air" was used in the treatment of typhus fever.

In one of these essays upon "The Influence of Trades, Professions and Occupations in the United States on the Production of Disease," the author shows clearly how the crowding together of children in the tenement districts produces gastrointestinal disease and death, proving that at this distant period the virtue of fresh air was appreciated.

In 1850 to 1860 Dr. Clarke treated a very large number of cases of typhus fever in Bellevue Hospital by the fresh air method. The windows were removed; in winter stoves were placed before the open spaces to insure a slight heating of the air, but the patients were given the fresh air treatment, as we understand it in the fullest sense to-day. The results were vastly superior, the death rate very markedly lower than the mortality among the same class of patients in the same hospital at the same period in the hands of the other members of the staff where fresh air was not used. It is a well-known fact that in times of war patients treated with fresh air in tents always do better than those confined in hospitals.

The phenomena of child life have often occupied the attention of psychologists, and new theories are formed every day for children by educators. Theoretically, they are making the super-child, soon to be the father of the superman. We, however, should be quite content if parents can be taught to appreciate the advantages accruing to the child from correct feeding, combined with fresh air and the influence they exert upon the mental and physical development of the growing child.

Everyone should be made to understand how important it is for the very young to be taught how to stand, lie down and sit properly, and that deep breathing is the proper and only sure way to secure full lung expansion.

Let us all join hands and preach fresh air; vote for open squares, endorse roof gardens, have adenoids and tonsils removed, and if we are willing as a society to endorse and work for the fresh air treatment with the same zeal and enthusiasm as we have worked for fresh and pure milk, our results will be as great a success as has been secured by our milk enthusiasts.

A PLAN OF DEALING WITH ATROPHIC INFANTS AND CHILDREN.

BY HENRY DWIGHT CHAPIN, M.D.,
New York.

The problem of dealing with the sick and ailing infants of the poor must occasion much thought to those who have worked a great deal with this class. The usual forms of charity intended for their relief consist in attendance at dispensaries, day nurseries, the visits of district physicians or nurses from dispensaries and settlements, the extending of hospital accommodations to proper cases and fresh-air excursions and homes in summer. But there is one disheartening feature that constantly confronts the worker who is seeking to permanently help these children, namely, their defective vitality from the wretched environment that so often surrounds them when returned to their homes.

They frequently pass from one institution to another, each one contributing its share of effort, but really not able to do more than temporarily relieve the most urgent necessities. These poor little waifs thus pass on from hand to hand until their waning vitality is exhausted.

It may be said that the fault really lies in deficient and inefficient fathers and mothers, and much of the trouble undoubtedly is here, but, even so, better measures of relief should be sought and will often yield results that are surprising if continued long enough.

All purely institutional work for these children should be only temporary. After acute illness has been relieved, they should have other management. If they must be sent back to faulty life conditions at home after discharge from an institution, the relief afforded by the latter will often be of very temporary value. Neither is good accomplished by sending them to other institutions, as the collecting of many little children under one roof is not good for them, no matter how well managed the institution.

After a long experience with this class of cases the writer has found that relief can be much better accomplished along the lines of family life with individual supervision instead of the collective life with institutional methods. Acting on this idea, the Speedwell Society was inaugurated in 1902, and has since been in successful operation. The plan followed is the boarding-out system, and the results have been remarkably good, considering that bottle-feeding has been exclusively employed, as wet nurses have never been available. The cases have been placed in carefully selected private families in the neighborhood of Morristown, N. J., which affords a very healthy location. A doctor and trained nurse have oversight of the cases. The foster mother is instructed in feeding and otherwise caring for the baby. A supervising nurse procures the children from the city and returns them to their homes when discharged from the care of the society, besides attending to many other necessary details of the work. She also endeavors to see that improved methods of care and feeding are carried on after the child is returned to its home.

The work of the society is not confined to the summer months. Children are received at any time of the year, and it is found that most valuable work can be done during the winter season. Neither is there any time limit for the keeping of the children. Each one is retained long enough to attain permanent improvement, or until it is proven that the case is hopeless. It is believed that it is better to permanently help a few than only temporarily to help many.

Most satisfactory results have been obtained in the cases of infants suffering from chronic malnutrition due to prolonged faulty care and feeding. In institutions, fed on the bottle, the vast majority of these cases will die, no matter how carefully they are nursed and fed. These babies should never be kept in institutions of any kind. The method of dealing with them should be changed. The experience of this society shows that, even on the bottle, a majority of them can be saved if a fairly good individual environment can be secured and careful oversight of the feeding maintained.

A hospital or institution of any kind should only serve as a temporary hold-up in cases of acute illness of infants, and they should always be sent out to recuperate after the acute symptoms have been relieved, and, if possible, to the country.

For the past six years the Speedwell Society has worked according to this method, with the following results: The first child was sent out March 19, 1902. The total number cared for from that date to March 19, 1908, is 817. The ages were as follows:—

Under three months 121
From three to six months 95
   "   six to twelve "   83
   "   one to two years 85
   "   two to five "   130
Over five years 303
                            —————
                            817

There have been 103 deaths at the following ages:—

Under three months 45
From three to six months 29
   "   six to twelve "   21
   "   one to two years 8
                            —————
                            103

The following were the causes of death:—

Marasmus or wasting 21
Gastroenteritis 45
Enterocolitis (chronic with malnutrition) 22
Bronchopneumonia 6
Acute lobar pneumonia 1
Tuberculosis 1
Diphtheria 1
Scarlet fever 1
Cholera infantum 1
Meningitis 2
Premature infants 2
                            —————
                            103

The results of the method, as judged by the number of deaths, may not seem very brilliant to those unaccustomed to deal with this class of cases. In glancing over the tables we see that a little over one-third of the cases under three months died; a little over one-quarter between three and six months, and one-quarter from six to twelve months died. After the age of one year there were only eight deaths among 518 cases. The heavy mortality among this class is under one year. This period is very hard to deal with in thin, badly nourished, bottle infants brought to institutions for relief.

The boarding-out method, under careful supervision in the country, is the best plan yet devised to relieve and save these infants. The first series of 121 cases would nearly all have died under ordinary methods of handling, and yet almost two-thirds of

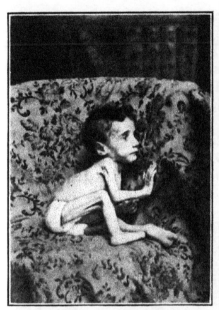 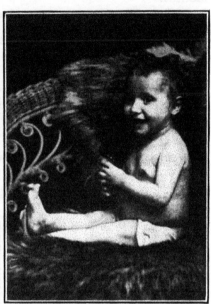

Condition May 18, 1905.   Condition September 8, 1905.

FIG. 1.—A case of extreme atrophy.

them were saved. They were poorly nourished from bad hygienic surroundings, with various degrees of digestive disturbance from faulty feeding on the bottle, and stationary or losing weight. A .arge proportion were restored to fair and even vigorous vitality, although kept on the bottle.

A larger proportion were saved from three to six months and from six months to one year—in the first series nearly three-quarters and the second series quite three-quarters being the proportion saved. These are brilliant results, considering that artificial feeding was still of necessity exclusively employed.

In some cases of marasmus the results have been really remarkable. As an example, Esther K., aged thirteen months, was sent out from hospital on May 18, 1905, weighing 9 pounds, 8 ounces. The extreme emaciation is shown in the picture. (Fig. 1.) She was returned on September 8, 1905, weighing 18 pounds, 8 ounces. In four months of this management she had doubled her weight and was a healthy, vigorous infant.

Morris R., three months; weight 5 pounds, 8 ounces—less than birth weight, and slowly but constantly losing. He was kept from January 19, 1903, to November 20, 1903, when he was returned, weighing 25 pounds—a gain of nearly 15 pounds in ten months.

Bessie M., fifteen months, weighed 14 pounds, 12 ounces on being received, November 22, 1905. She was sent back February 15, 1906, weighing 23 pounds. (Fig. 2.)

These cases are used as illustrations and are not so exceptional as might be supposed. They show that wasted infants can often be restored to proper vigor and development if handled in the way here proposed.

While wasting in infants is largely due to faulty diet in its inception and continuance, yet when the atrophy has proceeded to a certain extent the change to a proper diet is not usually sufficient to check the downward trend. These cases require, in

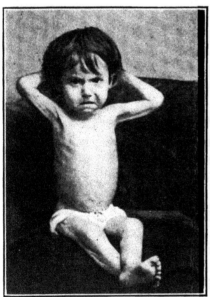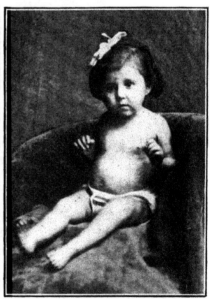

Condition November 22, 1905.   Condition February 15, 1906.

FIG. 2.—A case of atrophy with rickets.

addition, an altered environment that will furnish plenty of fresh air, good general hygiene and individual care. For this reason they never do well in institutions, no matter how carefully and scientifically they are fed. They cannot assimilate the best of food without an abundance of good air to assist in its oxidation;

oxygen is as necessary a food for them as proteid or fat. It is only individual housing and care with constant oversight that can accomplish good results.

In the work at Morristown twenty-four families have been employed. Some do better than others, and the doctor and nurse have them graded in their own minds as to their success and efficiency. Some of the foster mothers have been very successful in nursing feeble infants back to health, and take the greatest interest in the work. We aim to encourage them by praise, as the pecuniary reward—$12 per month—is small, but they feel they are engaged in a great undertaking. Some tire of the work, and others are dropped because of inefficiency. The tact and good judgment of the supervising matron are constantly called into play in retaining old homes that are satisfactory and in selecting new ones, but she knows the locality and the people, which is most necessary in such a work. Systematic, careful study of the field of operation is required if such a work is to succeed. Desultory, haphazard methods will not avail. The same care, routine and system that are usually brought to bear in institutional work must be applied here. There is nothing in common between the work of a well-organized society engaged in such an effort and the old-fashioned baby farming. The latter was justly abandoned, owing to the many abuses that sprang up in connection with it. In the Speedwell Society not more than one infant was placed in one family. Natural surroundings are thus insured and the danger of infection reduced to a minimum.

Briefly summarized, the plan that has worked well, and is advised in future dealing with neglected infants suffering from marasmus, comprises the following features:—

(1) Boarding out in a certain district of the country noted for its healthful conditions.

(2) Constant attention to diet and hygiene on the part of a doctor and nurse who are familiar with this class of cases and competent to deal with them.

(3) The infants are kept as long as necessary, until feeding is regulated and digestion and assimilation are improved sufficiently to result in an increase in weight. The work is continued during all seasons.

(4) The training up in a given neighborhood of a number of foster mothers, who, by constantly taking these infants into their homes, become expert in handling them under conditions

totally unlike those offered by the best institutions and far superior to them.

If such a plan is carried out, a large majority of these infants and children can be saved. No capital is required to be tied up in a building. The visiting doctor and nurse should be paid a salary, and outside of this, all the money given goes directly to the board of the children. If contributions fall off, the work is contracted until more comes in, when it again expands—resources and efforts thus acting automatically. The plan has been proven to be economically sound as well as practically efficient.

Every crowded community having much destitution can best look after its little waifs and strays and save most of them by arranging to board them out in a neighboring countryside under careful oversight, according to the method of the Speedwell Society.

DISCUSSION OF PAPERS BY DRS. NORTHRUP, GRAHAM AND CHAPIN.

AUGUSTUS CAILLÉ, M.D., New York.—I am in full harmony with everything expressed by the three essayists. Twenty years ago when I entered the babies' wards I tried to get the ladies in control there to understand the importance of cold fresh air to children, and some of them suggested that it was dangerous and that the babies would have to be boosted up with strychnia and other drugs. At the present time we have a roof garden, a part of which is covered and a part open, and a cold air ward, etc.

I endorse most emphatically the views of Drs. Northrup, Graham and Chapin. I believe that the breathing of cold fresh air is the most important therapeutic agent that we have.

A. JACOBI, M. D., New York.—I have been particularly interested in Dr. Chapin's paper. In the year 1870 I was a member of the medical staff of the Nursery and Child's Hospital, the pet institution of the elite ladyships of New York City. When I proposed boarding out infants and taking the curtains from the cribs, and when I proved that of 100 cases admitted to the hospital and retained there over three months 100 died, I was expelled from the institution. I was first told to resign, but I was correct in my views and told them that I was not of the resigning kind; that I would rather be expelled. They told my colleagues that if they did not expel me they would risk their own positions, and I was expelled by my own colleagues. We see how times change. I approve heartily of the endeavors of Dr. Chapin. He is a practical man and knows his business, and he has certainly been more successful than I was, perhaps because he is more circumspect.

There is a disease that has not been mentioned at all, a disease that fifty years ago we hardly knew in the United States. Since immigration and poverty have increased we have a great deal of it—I refer to rachitis. The disease is attributed by many to bad food. It is more due to bad air than to bad feeding. That is proved by the northern Russians and Swedes who have rachitis in their best families, because their winters are eight or nine months long and the babies are not removed from their close quarters. I had a patient about forty years ago, now one of the better known surgeons in New York, who had craniotabes; he had convulsions; he was at that time a child of seven or eight months. The only thing that saved him was our taking the baby away from the house and keeping him outdoors all winter. From the first hour the baby no longer had convulsions, and, in spite of his craniotabes, his brain was kept in such good condition and developed so well that now, not only is he a successful surgeon, but, what is more, he is a good doctor.

R. G. FREEMAN, M.D., New York.—As to measles, I would

relate two experiences. In the Nursery and Child's Hospital, in 1907, there were two epidemics, 71 cases and only 1 death. I think that is quite a remarkable showing. The second of these epidemics occurred while I was on duty and was a very severe one. We had a good deal of complicating otitis and a moderate number of complicating pneumonias. The whole ward afterward came down with bowel trouble, and it became necessary to make some change in what we were doing if we were to avoid a high mortality. It was in December, but the children were put out-doors and after that we had a rapid recovery from the diarrhea and no deaths at all. Later on, in March, I was on duty at the Foundling Hospital, where we had an epidemic of measles and scarlet fever. During this time cases of measles began to break out in the scarlet fever wards and there was no place to put them. Outside the ward was a closed piazza, and this we used for isolating these cases. All the measles cases were put out and they did remarkably well. One case had bronchopneumonia, starting with the measles, and that case did well too. So, I think, measles is very well treated by fresh air.

Dr. Jacobi said something that interested me very much as to the etiology of rachitis. I have felt convinced for some time that it was a disease of asphyxiation. The fact that it is a disease of cold climates and of winter; that they are worse in the spring and better in the fall; the failure in animal experiments to pro-duce the disease with different forms of feeding, and the fact that it occurs most remarkably in races accustomed to warm climates where they live out of doors, as the negroes and Italians, all point to this conclusion that it is a disease of bad air.

J. P. CROZER GRIFFITH, M.D., Philadelphia.—I would call at-tention to the fact that there is a difference in the way men use the term "fresh air," and that this leads to confusion sometimes, and I think this has done on this occasion. Among those speaking on this subject today three different things have been referred to under the term of "fresh air treatment," namely, the breathing of *fresh* air, the breathing of *cold* air, and the *exposure of the body* to cold air. It is evident that we are dealing with different conditions. When Dr. Northrup exposes a child with scarlet fever, having a temperature of 107°, to cold air to reduce the temperature, it is manifestly a very different thing from plac-ing a patient on a roof garden to breathe fresh air. So, too, when an authority is quoted to the effect that children in the first few months of life bear cold air badly, it is manifest that reference is made to the *chilling* by cold air, not the *breathing* of cold air. Whether or not the exposure to cold air for the sake of reducing hyperpyrexia is to be recommended—and I see no reason against it—there can scarcely be any discussion as to the advisability of having sick children breathe fresh air, whether warm or cool. As to the possible danger which may come from the exposure of the body to cold air, which the breathing of cold air might necessitate, that would seem to depend largely upon the nature of the disease. We all realize the difficulty or impossibility of giving a child a cold while it has fever. On the other hand, none of us would expose a very young marantic child in a cold room and take the covers off of it.

E. M. BUCKINGHAM, M.D., Boston.—The last speaker said what I was about to say, only much better than I could have said it.

It is a clinical fact that certain hospital pneumonias with dyspnea are given oxygen in the common way without relief, but are relieved when their beds are placed in the open air out of the wind.

C. B. PUTNAM, M.D., Boston.—For the last thirty-five years I have been connected with the Massachusetts Infant Asylum. When I first went in they were just beginning to farm out a few of the children. Since then this has developed to such an extent that of 125 patients less than 25 are kept in the hospital. The rest are boarded out in the country and there has been a remarkable reduction in mortality. The hospital is used partly for those who come in in an emaciated condition and need special nursing and partly for those who get sick while in. We find some cases suited for hospital care a part of the time.

L. E. LaFÉTRA, M.D., New York.—Just a word in regard to the objections made to the treatment in private practice. These can often be overcome by using the inside awnings or window tents, which allow the child to breathe the fresh air without being exposed. We have learned to do this in the treatment of tuberculosis and I find that it is very satisfactory.

CHARLES G. KERLEY, M.D., New York.—Typhoid is a disease in which I have been particularly interested with respect to this fresh air form of treatment. I have had very little trouble in applying the treatment in private practice. In fact, I have been surprised at the readiness with which intelligent people take it up. The people are prepared and ready; they have been made so by the plans for the treatment of tuberculosis.

I think Dr. Chapin's paper is most excellent; he has struck the key note of the management of these cases of atrophic infants, and if I were to say anything it would be to simply repeat what he has said with greater emphasis.

There is one point relating to the remarks of Dr. Jacobi and Dr. Freeman with reference to rachitis. No doubt oxygen deficiency has much to do with it, but you give the baby a good breast full of milk when he wants it, of a good character, and he will stand oxygen in sufficiency. Put them on the bottle, give them poor food, badly prepared, and you will get rickets. You get it under bad hygienic conditions quicker, of course, but you also get it under the best conditions. I still believe it is a nutritional disorder *per se.*

SAMUEL S. ADAMS, M.D., Washington.—We must draw a distinction between the methods of farming out babies in the time of which Dr. Jacobi speaks and the present time. The present-day method is backed up by means and intelligence; by means that can buy intelligence. They can afford to have competent nurses and skilled physicians. They do not simply board them out, as they did in those days, to some darkey with five or six children who, as I have often seen, would bring them to the hospital surprised that they could not keep "pot-liquor" on the stomach. Now in my city we have a Board of Charities, a board of children's guardians, who watch over the children and they are better supervised. They only give a limited number of children to one person to be cared for.

In regard to the fresh air treatment I have gotten as good results as those mentioned and have been surprised how even the ignorant show a willingness to carry out this treatment. To illustrate this an incident occurred recently; I was called in consultation to see a case in an Irish locality known as "Holy Hill." When I went up to the house the doctor said, "I know what you are going to suggest, but it will not do up here." The child was in a room 10 x 12, with the usual stove, cat and dog, and coal-oil lamp and there were about twenty people in the two rooms. The child, eighteen months old, was lying on a sofa with a temperature of 106° and evidently in a dying condition. I suggested to them that the child would die if kept where it was and that it might possibly be saved if the mother would take it upstairs, wrap up well and sit by the open window with it all night. She said she would. The doctor said he knew she would not and advised me not to be seen in that neighborhood for the next thirty days. Three or four days afterward I inquired about the child and was told that they couldn't get the woman away from the window and that the baby was living and doing well.

F. S. CHURCHILL, M.D., Chicago.—I think people are very ready to carry out this treatment much more willingly than the profession at large think. This is true not only among intelligent people, but among all classes. I have no difficulty whatever in private practice. In my dispensary practice I have had great assistance by having one of the nurses of the Visiting Nurse Association follow up the cases, going directly into the homes and looking after them.

P. J. EATON, M.D., Pittsburg.—The question of the adaptability of the nurse has much to do with it. Dr. Northrup's famous paper, entitled "23," gave me the inspiration to teach the fresh-air treatment to nurses. I lecture to nurses in four different hospitals and I have found that since giving them such instructions we have a much better chance with the treatment. We now have a corps of nurses who carry out intelligently what we desire along this line.

J. LOVETT MORSE, M.D., Boston.—We have heard a good deal today about fresh air and cold air for sick babies. I only want to remark that they do no harm to well ones.

A. JACOBI, M.D., New York.—Dr. Adams has suggested that the time of which I spoke was different from the present time—that a good deal of my ill success must have been due to that circumstance—but I beg to remind him of the fact that it is hardly forty years ago and at that time a good many of the principles of good infant feeding were known. I taught the same thing at that time that I still teach and which has proved so successful, and there are a good many of my pupils and friends who have come to my way of thinking. So that these babies appear to have been fed correctly. Moreover, the tendency was at that time not to send the babies out with a negro nurse, in droves, but to send them out one by one to farmhouses just as we are doing now. The Department of Charities had commenced for several years to board out children one by one, and if the example had been followed everything would have been well, but at that time it was the wish, as it always is of people in power, and ladies particularly, to control as many subjects as possible, and they wanted everyone under their roof, and they had to bury everyone. As has been said to-day, that is the result in institutions to-day, and it was then. I am glad to have lived long enough to know that common sense is beginning to prevail, and evidently it is prevailing, for Dr. Chapin has proved it today.

E. E. GRAHAM, M.D., Philadelphia (closing discussion).—I pointed out in my paper that in the early part of the nineteenth century it was appreciated by a few that fresh air was an absolute necessity. We have never had a foundling hospital in Philadelphia, and I think the reason is that in 1871 a number of prominent medical men and others got together and discussed the advisability of erecting one. Dr. Jacobi was quoted at that meeting in 1871 as being decidedly opposed to the foundling hospitals, and the records of the foundling hospital in New York, where such a large percentage of children died, were brought up. At that meeting the idea suggested by Dr. Chapin to-day, of farming out, as they called it then, was advocated. In other words, what we are discussing to-day has been talked about for nearly a century, and boarding out, as suggested by Dr. Jacobi and such as was the unanimous verdict of these medical and legal men was endorsed then. These methods have been practiced by a few men for a great many years, but it seems to me that we are only now beginning to get out ourselves and preach it. If we as a body will be as enthusiastic about this matter of boarding out children and the securing for them of fresh air as we were in our campaign for pure milk we will get excellent results.

WILLIAM P. NORTHRUP, M.D., New York (closing discussion).—I would emphasize a point that Dr. Graham has mentioned: that we have raised the standard of quality of milk. Now, by paying equal attention to this other hygienic measure, we will bring it into more prominence and greater usefulness. See what has been done in creating a better quality of drinking water by agitating the matter. Air is too cheap; we do not appreciate things until there is a dearth of them.

Dr. Griffith has raised the point that we were not definite enough in our phraseology. I have purposely made my talks concerning pneumonia and its treatment in the open air. If pneumonia can be successfully treated in the open air, other acute infectious diseases certainly can. I think the body breathes the air and needs the stimulus as much as the lungs.

As to typhoid, I am not at all sure that cold air will take the place of the bath. I have tried it a little, but have not had an opportunity to try it enough.

An old pal of Dr. Jacobi's, Dr. Oliver Wendell Holmes, said:
"God lent His creatures light and air and waters open to the
     skies;
 Man locks him in a stifling lair and wonders why his brother
     dies."

HENRY D. CHAPIN, M. D., New York (closing discussion).—
I must say that I feel very deeply on this subject, as for many years I do not think I lived up to my light, and I do not believe many of us have. We have seen hundreds of these babies slip through our hands under the usual methods of treatment in institutions. I have had the best hospital wards, roof gardens, convalescent homes especially for these cases, and yet it was the same thing; every baby under one year of age did badly if kept long. History is repeating itself, and the time has come when we who are supposed to know something about this thing should speak, and in no uncertain manner.

With regard to the boarding-out system: the plan I follow is not simply farming out: it is putting them out in a restricted area of the country, with skillful doctors and trained nurses and with people who can be watched. There are all kinds of objections. Some said you will kill these children, but it is not true, and they will all do better in this way.

ACUTE POLIOMYELITIS (AN EPIDEMIC).

BY HENRY KOPLIK, M.D.,
New York.

The epidemic of so-called poliomyelitis, which visited New York last summer, was certainly not only the most extensive known in New York, but possibly in the United States. Something over 1,200 cases were reported to the New York City and State Boards of Health. The conditions of weather and of atmosphere were not unusual, and the writer of this reference was present in New York during the whole epidemic, and his experience includes a large number of cases seen in private office work and with other physicians. The disease was certainly, in its characteristics, an epidemic one. It was quite widely distributed, being limited particularly to the city limits, with a few scattering cases in the suburbs. It cannot be said that to any extent the cases occurred in the filthy or crowded portions of the city; I have heard of cases in Tuxedo, a fashionable suburb for city residents. There were cases in parts of Brooklyn in sparsely populated districts; cases in the Bronx, where the sanitary conditions among the poor are exceptionally good; and finally, I saw cases in the crowded and filthy portions of the city. The conditions of the streets were not unusual; they were about as clean as one can expect to find in a large, densely populated city. There was nothing in the water supply that attracted attention, and the milk supply was certainly as good, if not better, than in previous summers. Therefore, so far as external hygienic influences are concerned, the conditions were not better, and certainly not worse, than they have been in previous years; consequently, the local conditions causing the epidemic must remain a matter of speculation.

The epidemic, in its behavior and in the several cases seen by me, certainly resembled very closely what was seen by Harbitz in Sweden, and so classically described by him in his work on the pathological aspect of this question. As to the character of the disease, it affected children of all ages from earliest infancy to adolescence; and some cases occurred in adults, but they were few and scattering.

The general characteristics of the disease can in no way be said to resemble what has been classically understood to be poliomyelitis anterior, but it is rather a disease which hitherto has been unknown to us in many of its manifestations. Many of these cases at first resembled meningitis, and yet some of the physicians with whom I came in contact saw immediately that they were in the presence of something new, which was not meningitis, and at the same time in some cases presented many meningeal symptoms.

I think it will be best from a clinical standpoint to describe certain sets of cases which occurred in this epidemic of so-called poliomyelitis. First, there were the cerebral cases. In these cases a child in apparent health would either suddenly go into a condition of unconsciousness, or would go to bed perfectly well, awake with a febrile movement, vomiting and complaining of headache, then pass into a condition of sopor, or with a very bright sensorium would develop paralysis of all four extremities. If the case was an extreme one, the paralysis would suddenly be followed by increasing sopor, in which the patient suddenly developed symptoms referable to the bulb or enlargement of the medulla; there was difficulty in respiration due to paresis or paralysis of the respiratory muscles; difficulty in swallowing; the sopor increased to coma with increasing paralysis in some cases ending with the death of the patient apparently from respiratory failure and bulbar paralysis. In other cases these cerebral symptoms would abate and a mild condition of sopor would be replaced by a clear sensorium, but with complete paralysis of all four extremities. In some cases there would also be paralysis of the abdominal muscles, or paralysis of the thoracic muscles and abdominal muscles, and muscles of the back, in addition to the muscles of the four extremities. These patients would also show distinct signs of bulbar paralysis with a form of breathing which is purely diaphragmatic, that is, the abdomen at each respiration would be protruded, the thorax remaining inert.

In other cases a child would go to bed apparently well, and these are what I call the neuritic cases; they would awake with acute pains in the extremities, referred in many cases to the joints. So acute were these pains that the patients would cry out in the night, even if not disturbed. Gradually, in many of these cases, a paralysis of one or all of the extremities would develop with a clear sensorium. In these cases also, as in the first set of cases, there was a mild febrile movement. The temperature, which at first was quite high, would drop to near the normal or normal and stay at the normal or continue for a time with slight variations above the normal. These cases were often mistaken for rheumatism. In some, after having lasted for three or four weeks, the pains would subside and leave a paralysis either of both extremities, or one upper or one lower extremity, and in other cases there was nothing left to show that the patient had been completely paralyzed but a slight facial paralysis. Some of these cases, after having been watched through a course of months, certainly impressed one as similar to those mentioned by Harbitz and Strümpell as occurring in these epidemics, and I believe that many of these cases were purely neuritic. On no other ground can I explain the almost complete recovery of many of these cases; cases which were completely paralyzed for weeks, which suffered intense agony from neuritic pains would, after two or three months, walk into my office with nothing to show of the serious illness through which they had passed but a slight paralysis, possibly of the peronei muscles as evinced by a slight halt in the gait.

The third set of cases were those which we are accustomed to see at times in which there is no epidemic. Cases which correspond minutely to what has been described by Charcot and his pupils as acute poliomyelitis anterior. That is, a patient would go to bed completely well and awake with a paralysis of one or two extremities, varying as the case may be; or a paralysis of a little group of muscles, either in the arm, forearm, thigh, leg or face. Many of these cases of anterior poliomyelitis acted very much as the text-books tell us they ought; a slight disturbance of the stomach, a febrile movement which lasted for a day or so, to be followed by paralysis.

We have therefore three distinct sets of cases—the cerebral, the neuritic with paralysis, and the classical cases of anterior poliomyelitis. It is hard to say at this period whether the pathology of all of these cases was similar. It is certainly safe to say that they were all the victims of some infectious agent. The cerebral cases, of which some were fatal, were autopsied, two of them in my hospital service, which was then under the care of Dr. Henry Heiman. The pathological appearances, gross and microscopical, were identical in these fatal cases with what has been described by Harbitz. Some of these cerebral cases were punctured in the hope that something might be discovered in the cerebrospinal fluid which would give a clue to the affection. Some of the punctures were warranted by the presence of the cerebral symptoms simulating as they did very closely meningitis. Nothing was found but a polynuclear cytosis. No bacteria were found by culture.

I will not describe the appearances so beautifully related by Harbitz in his work, but anyone who is acquainted with the relation of these appearances must admit that they give us an entirely different picture from what was formerly described as characteristic of anterior poliomyelitis. The areas of softening and hemorrhages to be found in the brain and cord are certainly not characteristic of anterior poliomyelitis, so that the term "poliomyelitis" must be accepted as a temporary nomenclature when applied to these epidemic cases. It certainly does not give us any idea of the characteristic lesions in the epidemic fatal cases.

I assume that the pathology is known as described by Harbitz and will not dwell any longer on this part of my theme.

Speaking of the cerebral cases, the form of paralysis was certainly peculiar. If the patient was not unconscious the sensorium was clear, and still the patients were unable to lift the extremities or to help themselves. They seemed to lie as if in a trance, and this in the presence of an absolutely normal temperature, or very little above the normal. The neuritic cases, however, were peculiar in that they not only had pain in the extremities and joints, especially at night, but there was great hyperesthesia; the little ones cried out in protest whenever examinations were made. They were perfectly helpless at the time that these pains existed. They could not sit up and had to be carried. The recovery in many of these cases was so complete that the conclusion is inevitable that no lasting infection of the cord occurred, but rather that the affection was limited to the nerve trunks.

As to the reflexes: It is well known that the reflexes in anterior poliomyelitis, as we understand it, are absent. In the vast majority of these neuritic cases the reflexes were increased at the knee, and in some cases which resembled anterior poliomyelitis as we classically know it, the reflexes were present and not absent. In the cerebral cases the reflexes were obtained, but there was no Kernig sign nor Babinski reflexes.

What was especially astonishing in this epidemic was the rapid atrophy of muscle in those cases in which the paralysis was to remain permanent and the quick development within a week of the onset of the reactions of degeneration, and what was more startling, the contractures which occurred following very quickly the rapid atrophy of the muscle. In my own service, one case, which is still in the service, is impressive. This child developed the atrophy after being paralyzed in all four extremities in the arms, forearms and muscles of the hand to such an extent as to give us the classical picture within a very short period, two or three weeks, of Duchenne's paralysis. The lower extremities showed the rapid atrophy of the muscles.

As to recovery: I have mentioned those cases in which a complete paralysis of all four extremities was followed by as rapid a recovery of power, so as to leave but very little evidence of paralysis. This fortunate ending was not uncommon in some cases, and as I have intimated, it was especially evident in the neuritic cases. Other cases which presented a picture of anterior poliomyelitis with absolute paralysis and atrophy of the muscles, of one lower extremity, for example, made an absolute and complete recovery to an extent which is only occasionally seen with the sporadic form of the disease; that is, the recovery included all the muscles of the extremity, excepting an isolated group such as the peronei, and even in this group, only certain muscles were affected, so that the child within a few weeks recovered the use of a limb which had been absolutely paralyzed with very little atrophy to show that the affection had been present.

Some of the cases which had been completely paralyzed in all four extremities recovered so that they could walk, but the upper extremities remained absolutely paralyzed with the exception possibly of the power to lift the arms and forearms to a slight extent, with marked contractures. If a case recovered after having been paralyzed in all four extremities the Achilles muscles were very sharply contracted and demanded tenotomy within two months after the onset of the affection. After tenotomy was performed the patient was able to get about, of course, showing paralysis in other groups of muscles in the lower extremities.

At the Hospital for Deformities in New York there have been a series of cases of facial paralysis treated, which was the only evidence in this epidemic of the disease after the onset of fever and gastric disturbance. Many of these cases were mistaken for meningitis of a tuberculous variety, the temperature being low or normal. One such case I saw in my office that had been thus diagnosed, the child being otherwise perfectly normal, the fundus of the eye being normal, the ears also being normal, subsequent events proving the correctness of the diagnosis, inasmuch as the case I am speaking of made a complete recovery so far as the facial paralysis is concerned. In this case there was a slight concomitant paralysis of the deltoid, which improved.

As to the causation and the mode by which the infectious agent enters the system, I have two theories to offer. In the vast majority of the cases I have seen, and in fully 60 per cent. of those seen by Gibney in the Ruptured and Crippled Hospital, there was a history of some disturbance of the intestine. In many of my cases there was a distinct history of diarrhea, in others constipation. In another set of cases, especially those with neuritis, I found that there had been a distinct attack of tonsillitis, and in several of these cases a culture had actually been taken of the throat, and nothing found but streptococcus infection, so that I believe that through the tonsils and through the gut an infectious agent must have reached the general nervous system.

Our nomenclature of this disease will certainly have to be revised. We can scarcely now speak of this disease as poliomyelitis, nor can we exclude from this epidemic the cases which I have mentioned, which resembled very closely the classical cases of anterior poliomyelitis and the classical cases of acute infectious neuritis. In other words, here we have a new infectious agent which is capable of causing paralytic disturbances, even death, by affecting the gray matter not only of the cerebrum, the medulla and the thorax, but also the white matter and axis cylinder of the nerve trunks.

As to the prevalence of the cases which have passed through this epidemic and retained their paralysis and disabilities to any degree, it is certainly sad to see how many children have been incapacitated by this epidemic. In one small institution, the Hospital for Deformities, there are not less than 150 odd cases coming for constant treatment, cases which show all varieties of paralysis and contractures and disabilities. The treatment which has been pursued, and which seems to give as much aid to nature as pos-

sible in these cases, has been that so much pursued in other forms
of neuritis. Hot baths have given a great deal of comfort to the
little ones, varied by massage of the extremities. Electricity at
first seemed rather to aggravate the symptoms, especially in those
cases in which there was pain along the nerves, but subsequently,
after the acute symptoms had subsided, the electricity in the form
of the rapid alternating current seemed to help to tone up the
muscular apparatus.

In cases of complete paralysis I found that empirically I followed the old treatment in vogue at the time Charcot first described the affection; the intramuscular injection of strychnin
was given to most of the cases with complete paralysis, one injection a day in the heart of the group of muscles affected.
Whether this was of any utility it is difficult to say; but many of
the cases treated thus made a good recovery. Cupping along
the spine was tried in many of my cases as a matter of routine.
I cannot say that any treatment did good except that directed
toward the alleviation of the pain, and for this I found the anti-
rheumatic remedies of the coal tar series, such as aspirin, of decided utility.

"EARLY SYMPTOMS IN SIXTY-THREE CASES OF THE RECENT EPIDEMIC OF ANTERIOR POLIOMYELITIS."

BY L. E. LA FÉTRA, M.D.,

New York.

The ordinary conception of anterior poliomyelitis is that of a disease which begins with vomiting, fever and more or less general nervous irritability, occasionally convulsions and delirium. Within one or two days there is paralysis in one or more of the extremities. The text-book descriptions would make the diagnosis very simple because of the early appearance of paralysis and because of the lack of marked cerebral or nervous symptoms and the absence of pain, tenderness or of rigidity in the extremities.

The recent epidemic in New York and vicinity has furnished an opportunity to observe many cases whose symptoms do not agree with the ordinary conception of the disease and has therefore offered many a difficult problem in diagnosis. On this account it has seemed worth while to the writer to make a study of the early symptoms of 63 cases of the disease; of these 20 were under treatment at the Babies' Hospital, 40 were observed at the Children's Department of the Vanderbilt Clinic and 3 were private patients.

The *conditions preceding the onset* of the disease were not sufficiently uniform in any number of cases to justify any conclusion. Some of the suggestive histories are as follows:

Of the Babies' Hospital cases:—

Henry S., two and a half years old. Was taken for a long drive. Came home very tired. Had fever that night and for six days following. Was paralyzed in both extremities on the morning following the drive.

Arthur D., three and one-half years old. Had been vomiting every day from August 24th until September 1st. Was not considered ill although he had fever from 99° to 101° F. On the eighth day he was found to be paralyzed in both lower extremities.

Edmund J., three years old. Was in good health, the first

symptom being severe occipital pain. This lasted for five days and was accompanied by slight fever. Then it was noticed that he had a general weakness and was unable to stand although he could move the lower extremities.

Rose J., nineteen months old. Perfectly well, and had no vomiting, but fever and restlessness for one day when paralysis was noted in both upper and lower extremities. The fever continued for two days after the appearance of paralysis. There was in this case some rigidity of the neck, but no pain in the paralyzed limbs, the paralysis being flaccid. (This type of case where the patient was in apparent perfect health and was suddenly taken with fever and paralysis was very common throughout the series.)

Arthur F., two and one-quarter years old. Swallowed a penny on September 18th. Was given an active purgative. That night there was fever and drowsiness and weakness of the extremities was noticed. On successive days the legs were paralyzed, the arms were very weak, and finally on the third day showed distinct paralysis.

John L., one year old. Had a cough and low fever for one week; then one morning paralysis was found in both lower extremities. There had been vomiting at the onset.

Sadie B., two years old. Was in apparently perfect health until she fell from bed. Walked a little for the next two days, but on the third day was unable to walk and it was found that she had paralysis of the left arm and leg.

Charles W., thirteen months old. Was apparently well until he fell from a low chair. When picked up it was found that the whole left upper extremity was paralyzed.

Among the Vanderbilt Clinic histories the following were noteworthy:—

Rachel F., thirteen months old. Was apathetic and somnolent for one week; was then in a stupor for forty-eight hours; then she became irritable and had an attack of vomiting with fever. There was rigidity of the neck, and on the day after vomiting it was found that both upper and both lower extremities and the left side of the face were paralyzed. There were pains in the limbs early, along the peripheral nerves, in the muscles and apparently also in the joints. Both legs and arms were said to be swollen. The case terminated in complete functional recovery, except in the left arm, forearms and left side of face.

George C., one and one-half years old. Had a high fever up to 105°F., lasting one week, but without any initial vomiting. There was restlessness and delirium. Four days after onset the arms were paralyzed; next the muscles of the back and finally the legs, all within the first week. The muscles of the abdomen were next affected so that the abdomen was distended. There was no pain or tenderness in the limbs and no rigidity of the neck.

Ralph C., two and one-half years old. Had cough and fever for three days. He kept complaining of pain in the left leg and a sensation of prickling. The paralysis was flaccid and recovery complete.

Eleanor B., six and one-half years old. Felt pain in back of neck on Saturday. On Sunday she walked with difficulty and had a temperature of 101°-102° F. On Monday she could not walk at all because of paralysis in left foot and leg.

David S., three years old. Had fever, pain and rigidity of the back and of the neck. The next day there was paralysis of both legs. For two days he was unable to urinate and there was constipation for three days. There was general painfulness of limbs, including the joints and the muscles.

Nellie S., ten months old. A nursing baby. Had fever, slight vomiting, convulsions and coma. Paralysis appeared two days after onset. For two weeks it was necessary to catheterize the baby. There was paralysis of both upper extremities and of both legs.

Ethel H., six years old. Had been trolley riding and had eaten various kinds of refreshments. That evening she vomited and had high fever. In twenty-four hours there was rigid paralysis of the left thigh, leg and foot. Both legs were painful, the muscles of the left leg being especially so. There was no rigidity of the neck.

Among the 3 private cases 2 are worthy of mention:—

Baby T., A little girl ten months old. She had a disordered digestion with fever up to 101°F., vomiting and great restlessness. In four days she had gradually sunk into a stupor which lasted for three days. She could be roused, but lay very still. The temperature after onset was not over 102⅜°F. Her pulse and respiration were irregular, the latter suggesting Cheyne-Stokes. The fontanel was not bulging, there was no Kernig's sign, and the extremities were flaccid; reflexes normal. On account of the stupor and the irregularity of pulse and respiration, the question of tuberculous meningitis arose, but because of the lack of rigidity of the neck or bulging of the fontanel it was decided to wait a few days before making lumbar puncture. Paralysis of both legs and of the right arm developed in four days and the baby's mind became clear at about the same time.

S. E. J., nine-year-old boy. On September 22d, after a very good summer at Lake George, the boy returned to New York. Had examination at school the following day and went to school on September 25th. On September 26th, after playing in the park for an hour and a half, he became tired and sat on a large stone watching a fire for about an hour. When he went home he was quite tired but seemingly well. That night he was very restless and complained of pain in stomach, although nothing unusual had been eaten. The next morning, September 27th, he had some headache, pain in both eyes, and slight aching throughout body. The right eye was red and there was some lacrymation. His temperature was found to be 101, and there was a little redness of the throat. He was kept in bed all day and had a good sleep that night. The next day, September 28th, he felt well so that he went to the country for over Sunday, taking a railroad trip of four hours. He returned to town on September 30th and seemed well the next day, so that he went to school (October 1st). At noon, when his mother went for him, he complained that he could not walk home because he had such a stomach ache and because his eyes pained him on coming out into the light. He walked half a dozen blocks and then began to cry because of pain in the eyes. He sat down on a bench and his hands and feet became cold, although he did not have real chill. After coming home in the street car he went to bed and did not care for any luncheon. When seen by me at five o'clock he had intense headache, photophobia, pain on movement of the eyes and pain on movement of the limbs. The temperature was 101°F., later mounting to 102°F. The tendon reflexes were all tested at this time without any changes being noted. There was no nausea nor vomiting during the night, but he complained bitterly of pain, mostly in the head. The next afternoon the symptoms were exaggerated, and there was, in addition, pain in the back and neck and stiffness of the neck. Dr. Holt saw the boy in consultation that evening. Complete examination failed to give definite diagnosis. The next day the pain and rigidity in back of the neck were increased, and he was unable to walk, although there was no paralysis. There was, however, an increase of the pain in the extremities. The next day, October 2d, the temperature rose to 103°F. The painful rigidity of the limbs was marked. Dr. Holt saw the patient, and at this time 15 c.c. of clear fluid were drawn by lumbar puncture. The fluid was negative on examination. On October 5th the urine had to be drawn with a catheter, and this was necessary for three days. The rigidity and pain in the back of the neck lasted for nine days. The child developed partial paralysis of both upper and both lower extremities. Painful cramps in the arms and legs were a marked feature and the pain in the legs persisted for three and one-half weeks. The legs were held drawn up and flexed at the knees for two and one-half weeks. After the third week rapid improvement took place. The child spent the winter in Bermuda and has recently returned to New York able to walk without a crutch or brace. There is still some dragging of the right foot.

The peculiar features of this case were: First, the intermission at the onset, there being three days of apparent perfect health after probably what was the beginning of the disease. Second, the intense headache, photophobia, rigidity of the neck, and the peculiar cramping pains and tenderness of all the extremities. Third, the slow appearance of the paralysis.

The details of the more important early symptoms in the 63 cases are as follows:—

Vomiting.—This occurred in 25 cases. In 1 it lasted for six days. As a rule, it occurred only at the time of onset.

Constipation.—This was present in 14 cases; therefore not at all characteristic.

Diarrhea.—This occurred in 17 cases. It was severe, lasting for a week or more in 4 cases. In regard to this symptom it should be emphasized that the cases occurred during the midsummer, and that most of the patients that suffered from diarrhea were young children or infants. It does not seem significant.

Cough, tonsillitis or sore throat existed in only 6 cases.

Fever was noted as present in 52 of the cases. It was probably present in all. The range of the temperature was from 100°-102° F. in the milder cases and 101°-105° F. in the more severe. It lasted generally from two to three days, but in some cases more than a week.

Restlessness and Irritability were very common in this epidemic, being definitely noted as present in 37 of the cases. In 3 cases there was general hyperesthesia.

Delirium was present in only 2 of the cases.

Convulsions were present in 4 cases, being severe in only 1, and in that case being repeated for four times only through one day.

Rigidity of the Neck.—This was present in 11 cases; it was exceedingly painful and persisted for over a week in 1 case.

Tendon Reflexes.—So few cases were seen before the time of paralysis that the study of the reflexes at the onset was impossible. Of the 20 cases seen at the Babies' Hospital the reflexes were absent in the paralyzed limbs in 16 cases, the reaction was present but sluggish in 3 cases, and in 1 case it was present on one side, absent on the other, the paralysis involving both lower extremities. In 2 cases the patellar reflex was absent on both sides, while the paralysis involved only one lower extremity. In those cases where the paralysis was rigid the reflexes were not obtainable and in no case of the whole series was the tendon reflex found to be exaggerated. Babinski's sign was present in 3 of the Babies' Hospital cases, one of these being on the side opposite the paralysis.

Apathy was present in 10 cases. In all but one it occurred early in the disease.

Stupor was present in 4 cases, in one instance lasting for forty-eight hours and in another for three days.

Headache was noted as present in 10 cases, being general in 3, frontal in 5, in one of which it was very excruciating, and occipital in 2 cases.

Photophobia was definitely present in 3 cases.

Pain and tenderness in the affected limbs was present in 32 cases; also along the peripheral nerves in 2 cases, in the muscles in 5 cases, and on movement of the joints in 4 cases. This symptom should be emphasized, because it has rarely been noticed in sporadic cases and was an element in confusing the diagnosis with cerebrospinal meningitis and with neuritis.

Character of the Paralysis.—The paralyzed limb was flaccid in 58 cases, spastic or rigid in 5 cases.

The paralysis came on early in a large proportion of the cases; on the first day in 24 cases, on the second day in 9 cases, on the third day in 3 cases, and after two weeks or more in 4 cases.

Other Symptoms.—The left side of the face was involved in a case which had paralysis of both upper and both lower extremities. The muscles of both the back and abdomen were involved in 1 case. The muscles of the neck and of the larynx were involved in 1 case. The respiration and pulse were irregular in 1 case. There was partial paralysis of the bladder in 4 cases, a catheter being necessary for two to seven days in 2 of these cases. Opisthotonos existed for five days in 1 case and for ten days in another. There was general anesthesia in 1 case and hyperidrosis in 1 case. There were 2 cases of unilateral paralysis of the oblique abdominal muscles, resulting in one-sided bulging of the abdomen at the semilunar line.

Lumbar Puncture.—This was done in 14 cases, 13 of them being those at the Babies' Hospital. From 15 to 70 c.c. of fluid was removed. It was under no pressure in 4 cases, slight pressure in 5, and increased pressure in 5 cases. Fluid was clear in every instance and was negative for bacteria both by smear and culture. In only 1 case were any cells found, and in this instance there were a few mononuclears present.

Blood Examinations.—Counts of the white cells were made in only 6 of the cases, the number ranging from 13,400 to 20,600. In the severest case which terminated fatally, and in which the paralysis was very widespread, the white cells were 18,200.

The explanation of the irritative symptoms, such as pain, cramps, rigidity, photophobia, etc., is an interesting question. Harbitz and Scheele would explain these symptoms as due to the irritation of the peripheral nerves resulting from inflammation of the pia mater of the cord and brain, which they found in their studies. They believe that this infiltration of the pia always precedes the inflammation of the grey matter of the cord or of the cortex. They found no inflammation of the peripheral nerves.

The diagnosis of the disease in the beginning of the epidemic may be very difficult. This has been noted many times, the confusion with acute meningitis, as well as with multiple neuritis, being very easy when the irritative symptoms are pronounced. The liability of mistake in diagnosis was especially commented upon by Harbitz in his report of the Norway epidemic of 1903-

1906. It was also noted by Caverley, by Mackenzie and by Chapin in their reports of epidemics in this country.

The careful studies that have come from Norway and Sweden in the last few years, particularly those of Medin, of Harbitz and Scheele, and recently of Wickman, have shed new light upon this disease and upon other nervous disorders closely related. Medin found, alongside typical cases of spinal poliomyelitis, cases of poliomyelitis of the bulb—pontine encephalitis—and also cases of local cerebral spastic paralysis due to encephalitis. The epidemic of 1905 showed also a meningitic, a polyneuritic and an abortive form in which there was no paralysis. Cases of progressive paralysis—ascending or descending—were also seen.

On account of the existence of these types of trouble in the same epidemic, and on account of their all having essentially the same pathological basis, Wickman has proposed to group them all under the name of the Heine-Medin Disease. This disease he would classify as appearing under eight different forms, as follows:—

(1) Ordinary spinal paralysis; anterior poliomyelitis. (2) Progressive paralysis, usually ascending, less often descending; Landry's paralysis. (3) Bulbar paralysis; polioencephalitis of pons. (4) Acute encephalitis, giving spastic mono, or hemiplegia. (5) Ataxic form. (6) Polyneuritis, multiple neuritic type. (7) Meningitic form. (8) Abortive.

I have not attempted to classify my cases under these types.

Although most writers mention the fact that cerebral symptoms, such as convulsions or stupor, may be present, and also that painful peripheral irritative symptoms may occur, still the medical profession at large needs to have these facts emphasized in the interest of early diagnosis and proper early treatment.

DISCUSSION OF PAPERS BY DRS. KOPLIK AND LA FÉTRA.

DR. HOLT.—In regard to the question of the epidemic I think something additional might be said. It is now being studied by a committee appointed by several of the societies, and according to the best information that the secretary has been able to get the number of cases in New York is not far from 3,000. If that is approximately correct, it is not only the largest epidemic of the United States, but of the world.

During the fall and summer I saw a good many cases in the neighborhood of New York City and should not agree with Dr. Koplik that it was limited to New York City, though it occurred in much larger numbers in the city districts.

A thing that struck me was the groups of cases occurring together. A physician, now a candidate for membership in this Society, came home with his two children and within ten days of his arrival in New York both children came down with symptoms of the disease. Both were paralyzed and both recovered completely. We had at the Babies' Hospital a child admitted from a small home in a neighboring village, and in seven days from that a second child came down who had been sleeping in the same bed with this one. In Pleasantville a child was taken ill on Saturday, and the following Saturday his little brother came down with an attack. I was furnished with a report of cases with five or six occurring in the same family, or separated by a four or five days' interval. One, a woman who went to visit a friend whose child was suffering with the disease and her boy was placed in the same crib; three days later this child came down with the disease and was paralyzed. These coincidences were so numerous that they make a very probable showing for a mild degree of contagiousness in this form of the disease. I think we must admit that this disease belongs in the category of acute infectious diseases of the central nervous system, with possibly a mild degree of contagiousness behind it.

One of the striking things was the number of cases that recovered, and completely. Another is the number that died. We have been accustomed to look upon poliomyelitis as a disease with no danger to life. We had 3 fatal cases in the Babies' Hospital. The total mortality was something like 12 per cent. When death occurs in the sporadic form it is probably ascribed to something else than poliomyelitis.

Another striking thing which occurred in the epidemic was that the disease stopped with the advent of the month of October. That has been the history of the epidemics everywhere—that they have ceased with the beginning of cold weather. Whether it will occur again in New York next year we do not of course know, but it has been the history of the disease that it has recurred in this way.

Now with reference to the punctures and the results. The fluids from the Babies' Hospital were sent to the Rockefeller Institute and studied by Dr. Flexner with negative results from every point of view. Dr. Flexner thought that the findings somewhat opposed the view that there was an acute microbic infection of the spinal cord and the results suggested rather a toxic degeneration of the cord due to toxines produced somewhere else in the body.

Obstinate constipation was a symptom of several cases I saw, like the obstipation we see in some forms of disease. I have seen lately 1 or 2 cases of polioencephalitis which ran a course very much like the familiar picture of poliomyelitis. The children came into the hospital with a history of convulsions and developed stupor, but we soon saw that it was not meningitis. There were mental symptoms: the temperature would rise to 104 and then drop to normal. They recovered completely. In spite of the location of the disease, its onset, and febrile reaction were very similar to our spinal cases, except that the symptoms were entirely cerebral.

It suggests that we have a disease that is perhaps an acute inflammation of the central nervous system, which generally localizes its effects upon the anterior horns, but may affect the cerebrum without affecting the cord at all.

DR. JACOBI.—I have only a few words to say. It has been suggested by Dr. Koplik that because the disease shows so many different forms it must be something absolutely new. I cannot agree with that. There are many different types of the disease that have been observed. I believe if we refer to the last remark made by Dr. Holt we have it all in a nutshell. It is a disease of the nervous system, perhaps not of the cord itself, but of the whole central nervous system. We do not know the cause, but we know one symptom that is common; that is hemorrhages—small hemorrhages. They have been found, not only in the anterior columns of the cord, but also in the posterior; and, not only in the cord, but in the brain. According to their localization they will produce a number of different symptoms. It is not necessary that small hemorrhages should give rise to any symptoms whatever, at least as far as sensation, motion and intellect are concerned. We know that we have hundreds of little hemorrhages in cases of concussion of the brain which get well. In those cases we are not astonished at all to find no symptoms. They get well without paralysis or disturbances of sensation or intellect. A large number of such localized small hemorrhages in poliomyelitis or polioencephalitis may produce no symptoms whatever and leave no symptoms. It depends on the location as to how temporary or how permanent the symptoms will be. It appears to me that the character of the disease this year in a large majority of cases is more that of polioencephalitis than poliomyelitis. That explains a number of symptoms that formerly were not very common. We should remember that where polioencephalitis is predominating there should be intact patella reflex. In the cases where the cord is affected the reflex disappears in a very short time and atrophy will set in very soon. If we remember what we knew formerly of poliomyelitis, and that this winter the epidemic was twenty times as extensive as the largest of those that had been observed anywhere and the cases a hundred times as numerous as occurred in many of the epidemics, we should hesitate a little in demanding the same symptoms that were observed at that time, in those cases, that it was our lot to see last year. I would fall back upon the old reports—those of Heine in 1840 and 1860. Most all of his cases were of a different description altogether. He reported cases of children put to bed well and taken up paralyzed; nothing the matter with them at night and in the morning paraplegia. A number of cases, however, were reported by him in which there was the occurrence of fever in the night and paralysis in the morning. There were other cases in which the babies were sick in bed with, for instance, scarlet fever or pneumonia, and when taken from the bed it was found that they were paralyzed. So there were a number of different types even then. These are the cases and types which I have often seen, and described these nearly fifty years. Therefore, we should not be so astonished to find in an epidemic that is a hundred times as large as those were that there should be a number of different symptoms. We should be satisfied in saying, as we do not know the etiology, that it is a disease striking the nervous system as a whole, more in this place or that, as the case may be. Cases of polioencephalitis have a greater tendency to get well completely than cases of poliomyelitis. The latter get better frequently; well, entirely well, quite rarely.

Dr. Abt.—Were there any autopsies on the fatal cases, and what were the findings?

Dr. Kerley.—I had an opportunity to see in this New York epidemic 43 cases: 13 in the Babies' Hospital, 9 in other institutions, 3 in my own practice and 18 in consultation. I came into these cases late in August and early in September. The cases increased until October and then practically ceased.

Dr. Koplik and Dr. La Fétra have given such an admirable exposition of the symptomatology that I have little to say. I thoroughly agree with what Dr. Koplik says. I have seen more or less poliomyelitis for twenty years and I think in this epidemic we have had an entirely new proposition. In some of the cases it was absolutely impossible to differentiate between them and cerebrospinal meningitis. The rapid onset, retraction of the neck, stupor, etc.. was marked. Kernig's sign was ruled out in many of the cases because there was so much tenderness.

As to the territory of the epidemic, I found that the northern boundary was at Malden. There, with only twelve or fifteen children in the school, they had four with poliomyelitis. That would seem to be the apex of a triangle which extended down the river until it reached New York. The area was, as Dr. Holt has said, of very wide distribution.

One of the cases was particularly interesting to me: the child came down with acute symptoms of fever and vomiting and developed facial paralysis, the only evidence of paralysis that occurred and it persists at the present time. Evidently there was a nuclear involvement.

DR. MORSE.—I recently had occasion to analyze the cases of infantile paralysis which I had seen. Only three or four of them were seen last autumn. The results of this analysis, as will be seen, show that the type of the disease in the sporadic cases is essentially the same as during the recent epidemic in New York. Pain and tenderness were present in two-thirds of the cases, in some at the onset, in others beginning after two or three days; the duration was usually but a few days, but they sometimes persisted for a month. They were most often in the neck, but were sometimes general, usually in the affected portions. Tenderness over the nerve trunks, especially the sciatics, was not uncommon, and in some cases obscured the diagnosis.

Cerebral and meningeal symptoms were also common. In some, delirium and stupor persisted for several days. In 1 case stupor persisted for a week. Nervous irritability was also very marked in a number of cases. Headache was the first symptom in 1 case and persisted for several days. It preceded the paralysis and other symptoms by thirty-six hours. Rigidity, retraction and tenderness in the neck were not at all uncommon. They appeared, as a rule, on the second or third day, but were sometimes present at the onset. They usually disappeared after a few days, but sometimes lasted one or two weeks. The blood, during the acute stages, showed a leukocytosis.

DR. KOPLIK (closing discussion).—As to the postmortem findings, in 2 fatal cases at the Mount Sinai Hospital there were autopsies, the findings of which will be published later. In a general way they corresponded closely to what has been described here this evening; areas of softening throughout the cortex; areas of hemorrhage throughout the cord, and areas of softening in the cord. The opinion of Harbitz was confirmed that the disease begins in the meninges and extends from there.

This disease does not affect any other nervous disease that may be in progress at the same time. I saw a case, just before leaving:

a child came to me in March with symptoms pointing to some general nervous trouble; he felt tired and did not feel like walking; when he sat down he did not care to get up. A positive diagnosis was not made at that time. The child went through the epidemic and developed poliomyelitis and came into my office with paralysis of right upper extremity and also with pseudohypertrophic paralysis fully developed. The course of this child's nervous affection, which was perhaps more serious than the poliomyelitis, was not affected by the latter, and the two nervous diseases existed side by side.

THE NEED OF POST-GRADUATE INSTRUCTION IN PEDIATRICS.

BY AUGUSTUS CAILLÉ, M.D.,

New York.

In the making of a medical practitioner there is still a lack of system and uniformity, which is difficult to explain, except as we view it as one of the forms of inherited or transmitted human inertia noticeable along sanitary lines in general.

At the present time the best results are probably obtained where a student, endowed with good "preliminaries," enters a medical school which is part and parcel of a large university so located as to be able to offer to the senior student in medicine ample hospital facilities and abundant clinical material; with its curriculum so arranged that the undergraduate's time is not taken up by didactic lectures, and the student is early brought into contact with the evidence of nature's manifestations in health and disease by means of practical courses in chemical, physiological and pathological laboratories.

Small medical colleges can, no doubt, also turn out good practitioners on account of the greater care given to each student, but to accomplish this they must offer a system of "object lesson teaching," by means of which, as Agassiz tersely says, "One may study nature, not books."

Faulty as it is, we must confess that the wholesome impetus of a good medical school makes the student eager for the two years' hospital and bedside training which is to follow, and at the end of which he is fairly well equipped to be let loose upon the public as a general practitioner.

In the realm of pediatrics, however, the young physician, as he starts out upon his life of service, is deplorably ignorant. He may be able successfully to cope with difficulties in diagnosis and to formulate indications for treatment, and even carry out proper treatment in the adult, but when he is confronted with the problems presenting themselves as regards the hygienic, dietetic and specific management of the ailing child, he stands, as far as practical knowledge goes, *"vis à vis de rien,"* and is unable to stake and prove his claim in pediatrics unless he has had the very exceptional good fortune to have spent half a year in a hospital devoted to diseases in children.

During a twenty years' service as teacher in pediatrics, the writer has not met a single young hospital graduate other than ex-internes of a children's hospital, who, on inquiry, did not freely admit his lack of practical knowledge regarding a line of professional work which makes up one-half the practice of the family physician. It is evident, therefore, that the present facilities for acquiring the knowledge necessary to combat preventable infantile sickness and mortality are totally inadequate and that more practical instruction along the lines indicated is urgently needed.

How best to meet the demand for practical post-graduate instruction in pediatrics has taxed the efforts of those devoted to this kind of work.

The value of a good post-graduate course lies in the fact that under guidance of competent teachers one may first see a patient in the *"dispensary,"* then in the *hospital ward,* where medical, operative or specialistic treatment is carried out in detail. One may examine the patient, study his "chart," examine blood, sputum, excreta, puncture 'fluids in the *laboratory,* and, if the patient dies, one may witness the autopsy and examine the specimens obtained.

Dispensary Clinics.—A large ambulatory service is the *sine qua non* feature of a good medical school. Dispensary work (apart from its value to the community) is excellent discipline for acquiring the art of making more or less accurate diagnoses and sharpening the power of observation.

Hospital Wards in Connection with the Clinical Laboratory.— The "wards" in connection with a clinical laboratory afford every facility for accurate study and proper treatment of patients. The course and termination of disease may be watched, and it is frequently possible to "prove the case" by transillumination, surgical procedure, or autopsy. The "wards" are available for illustrating and demonstrating methods of prophylaxis (ventilation, isolation, disinfection and protective inoculation), for diet kitchen work, palatable medication, for surgical, orthopedic and other manipulative or electrical therapy and for teaching physical diagnosis and diagnostic punctures.

Bedside Instruction.—Making rounds with a *large class of students* is of little value. To make bedside observation available for large classes, any one of the class should be allowed to visit the wards and examine patients and study their records during a set time of two or three hours daily and at a time in which there will be no serious interference with other clinics or other work. For purposes of bedside instruction the writer makes use of a diagnosis chart which was presented to this Society on a former occasion, which assists a student to go through a routine examination of any case assigned to him.

Amphitheatre clinics have their advantages and drawbacks. To utilize clinical material to the best possible advantage requires a large floor space for setting up ten to twelve tables for the simultaneous examination of as many patients. Demonstrable regionary lesions can be marked in colors on the skin of a patient or may be recorded by means of a chart. Not more than four matriculates should be invited to each table and, guided by competent instructors, should be given an opportunity to examine each case. After such demonstration *en masse* the students would take their seats and the teachers would proceed to point out the important differential diagnositc features and therapeutic indications in each case. Diagnostic punctures and manual methods of treatment, such as stomach and bowel irrigation, bathing, feeding by gavage, tapping the thorax, the abdomen, the spinal canal, intubation, removal of adenoids and tonsils, etc., can be demonstrated with advantage before a large class. The Lumiere color photograph is also available for clinical teaching.

The broadening influence of pediatric study has not been sufficiently emphasized and is probably underrated, but must be conceded as we realize how thoroughly the practice in diseases of children brings us into close touch with almost every other special line of medical work, including general surgery, the eye, ear, nose and throat specialties, orthopedics, skin diseases, etc.

Owing to the lack of flexibility in medical matters, much time will pass before medical schools will be properly equipped to teach practical pediatrics, but it is so ordained that all evils will in time work their own cure, and these few reflections are offered as a small contribution to the propaganda of adjustment.

AN INQUIRY INTO THE STATUS OF THE KINDERGARTEN.

ISAAC A. ABT, M.D.,

Chicago.

INTRODUCTION.

It was in the hope of throwing some light on the medical aspects of the Kindergarten question that the investigation, of which this paper is a report, was instituted. This investigation was begun without prejudice either for or against the system and purely in a spirit of inquiry, with a view to obtaining information on some of the vital questions which the physician is called upon to decide in daily contact with his patients.

It may be stated at the outset that there is no intention of offering a final solution of the various questions involved. The opinions received from sources of equal authority are so diverse as to render a positive conclusion impossible. Indeed, as the subject is developed it will be noted the results obtained are in a sense disappointing. Yet I feel that the views expressed are of sufficient interest and importance to warrant the presentation of this paper, in which both the pros and cons of the question will be impartially stated.

It is beyond the scope of this paper to enter into a detailed discussion of the philosophy of Froebel. Yet, a résumé of the history of the Kindergarten will, I think, not be amiss.

SOME POINTS ON THE PHILOSOPHY OF FROEBEL.*

The kindergarten had its origin with Froebel (1782 to 1852), whose Philosophy of Education is based upon abstract thought. His philosophy is in essential agreement with the philosophical system known as Idealism, which formed such an important part in the intellectual life of the Germany of his day. The ideas of Kant, Fichte, Schelling and Hegel had impressed themselves on the thought of the times. When Froebel had arrived at the age of serious reflection, he was influenced by the philosophy of his predecessors. The philosophic spirit of Idealism, under the spell of which Froebel lived and breathed,

---

* For this reference to Froebel's philosophy, I quote freely from a paper by John Angus MacVannel, Ph.D., Instructor in Education, Teachers' College Record, 1903.

attempted to unify the world and human life and its keynote was the grandeur and dignity of man.*

Froebel did not present educational thought which was altogether new. Like all human progress, it was evolved from previous knowledge. The germs of Froebel's thought may be found among the ancient philosophers. Socrates, Plato and Aristotle speculated in a mystical way concerning the deeper problems of life. Similar speculations struggled through the Middle Ages and found vigorous exponents in Luther, Bacon and Comenius. Kant began a movement which thought to discover the unity of all life, of nature and humanity in the Absolute Spirit. Hegel developed this thought into a system. Froebel was directly influenced by the philosophic teachings of Rousseau and Pestalozzi. He sought the latter as his teacher and supplemented his doctrines by making all educational work all sided and universal.†

As Pestalozzi owed his inspiration directly to Rousseau, so Froebel, sitting at the feet of Pestalozzi at Ifferton, received the message from the lips and the work of his great master.

Froebel's strict adherents believe that education is no mere empirical matter, but has its warrant deep in the very nature of the world. But the unbiased reader will at times encounter in his writings conclusions that seem unwarranted, and important questions that are not satisfactorily answered. It cannot be permanently our purpose to accept Froebel's system without qualification, or at least more adequate interpretation in the light of results of later science and experience. It is at the same time all important that the fundamental truths of his thought shall be rationally preserved and that in the process of its worn-out forms its vital essence and spirit shall neither be lost, nor even for a time impaired. As Green, of Oxford, said of the system of Hegel, so may we say of the system of Froebel, "It will all have to be done over again." Yet, in this very process of transformation, the fundamental character of his thought will be more fully recognized and its permanence more completely assured. Commenting on the philosophy of Froebel, Oppenheim says:

"His methods rested upon a foundation of keen observation, of love, fellowship and sympathy. But he knew very little of the reasons outside of metaphysical considerations for his course of work. In addition, there was a certain amount of lazy thought, of mysticism in his belief. He set up a sort of glorified child worship."

No account of kindergarten instruction would approach completeness without a reference to the basic principle of Froebel's teaching, namely, a consideration of what he termed "gifts."

Froebel's presentation of the subject of Gifts appears extremely complicated.‡ The subject is a composite of mysticism, symbolism, mathematics, ethics and religion. The gifts were intended to serve a two-fold purpose in the education of the child:—(1) to awaken his inner life to the perception of natural forces, and (2) to interpret the external world for him.

THE GIFTS.

The degree of isolation that obtains in the study of the gifts is directly due to the conception that they are materials of independent

---

* MacVannel, Teachers College Record, November, 1903.
† "Law of Childhood," by W. N. Hailmann, 1889. Alice B. Stockham & Co.
‡ For the subject matter referring to kindergarten gifts, I quote freely from a paper by Harriet Melissa Mills, Teachers College Record, November, 1904.

worth. The logical outcome of this isolation can be known through the study of kindergarten programmes and the actual demonstration of them in the kindergarten. It is the common practice in preparing an outline or programme to select a number of typical experiences from Froebel's "Mother Play," which are intended to initiate the child, through play, into his total environment. Correlated with these plays are songs, games and stories. The gifts are developed along independent lines in harmony with the prevailing notion, through long series of exercises that depend upon the logical sequence of form for their deepest significance.

The most notable effort in programme making and the one that has gained widest acceptance is the unpublished outline by Miss Susan Blow. The gifts in this outline are administered largely on the basis of form. They represent the subject-matter of exercises that in their initial steps concentrate upon some abstract notion inherent in the various gifts. In an address before the International Kindergarten Union, Miss Blow said: "The material used by the children for their productions has a geometric basis. Spheres, cubes, cylinders, squares, oblongs, triangles—indeed most geometric planes, and many geometric solids, thus become familiar to the little workers. Using them, the child comes to perceive them in all the objects around him. Numerical relations are also suggested, and thus is put into the little hands the mathematical key which unlocks the gates of inorganic nature."

Turning now to the prevailing practices in the kindergarten, a striking illustration is afforded of what it means to follow the lines of least resistance in the Froebel philosophy. The decision having once been made that the child has urgent need to know the formal aspects of material things, the next step is to supply this need through the use of gifts. This the Kindergartner may do by preparing her own series of exercises, or she may turn to the Gift Book or various manuals, and find the exercises ready to hand that will unlock to the child the "whole wide world of form and its elements of faces, corners and edges." Or, easier still, she may adopt outright a programme that must, because formulated by someone of large experience and insight, contain all the elements that child nature can need.

The formal programme also affords opportunities for building life forms; and naming the object and its uses becomes the subject of interesting conversation. For example, in an exercise with the fifth gift, the child builds a boat with cubes and triangular forms. The object is interesting because it touches life; but the practice of leading the child to a condition of awareness of the form built as a boat trapezoid crowds the exercise out of the range of the childish comprehension.

One of the fundamental characteristics of the fourth gift is contrast in dimension—length, breadth, height. These elements of dimension are permanently embodied in each of the eight bricks into which the cube is divided, and are made the point of departure for an indefinite variety of exercises that emphasize the relative position of the bricks as they are built into the three classes of exercises known as life, beauty and knowledge forms. These exercises may at the same time concentrate upon any one of the following ideas as the principal aim of the lesson, viz., divisions of the cube, enclosure of space, extension plays, surface movements, forms illustrating the laws of balance, illustrative lessons and geometric forms, of which there are at least thirty-two examples of square and oblong prisms. Each gift has its own peculiar principles and laws to be demonstrated through play exercises, and these—known only to the teacher—constitute the almost endless resources of the kindergarten gifts.

In kindergartens where the logical geometric sequence of the gifts is held inviolate, the children play through exercises that emphasize sphere, cube, cylinder, square and oblong. They count faces, corners and edges, first on the gifts and then on the objects around them.

They discover vertical, horizontal and oblique lines, angles and triangles of every description, while prisms—square, triangular, rhomboidal, trapezoidal, etc., are made to develop in logical progression; and the road to discovery is so hedged about with limitations and restrictions that no element of chance enters to prevent the prearranged achievements. For example, in developing the right angle two sticks are given to the child, and the impulsive response results in the perfectly natural discovery of the right angle. This procedure has been defined as the "method of restricted freedom."

It is a well-known fact that Froebel did not complete the series of gifts as they are used at the present time. He left many vague hints concerning the extension of the gifts by the addition of new forms—and subsequently of more sub-divisions—that would render the series more complete in its evolution of form, and further elucidate the fundamental properties of matter, time and space. There has been a persistent effort on the part of his followers to realize these suggestions, with varying success.

It is needless to say that as time has gone on the general adherence to the strict Froebelian teaching has relaxed, and while in some quarters there remains a semblance of orthodoxy, nevertheless, in the more enlightened quarters the interpretation is very liberal, and it would seem, almost at a glance, that the strict observances laid down by the founder must come to be regarded as obsolete because they are antiquated and not in accord with any definite knowledge of the brain perceptions of the child. The modern kindergartens, under the most enlightened leaders, tend to abandon the formal methods and programme and consider "that, after all, the child remains the heart and the inspiration of it all."

MANNER AND LIMITATIONS OF THE INVESTIGATION.

The investigation of kindergartens, from the physician's point of view, was suggested to me as a result of numerous conversations which I had with medical men concerning this subject. Some thoughtful colleagues were in the habit of advising parents most strenuously against sending children to kindergarten. Many of the reasons physicians gave for taking this position will appear in the subject matter which follows. I undertook the investigation in the hope of obtaining authoritative opinions. I myself could not arrive at any definite decision, nor was any conclusive information to be found in the medical literature. It seemed to me that in order to make the investigation far-reaching enough, it would be necessary to receive information from various sources. I therefore sent questionnaires to physicians located in various parts of the country. Opinions from those in leading positions in pediatrics and neurology were solicited. A similar blank was sent to educators. A different form of question blank was sent to kindergarten teachers and instructors in kindergarten colleges.

I wish that I might here give full credit to all those who replied to my inquiries, but space and time forbid, and I take this opportunity of extending my thanks to all who replied, assuring them of my appreciation of their co-operation, without which the preparation of this paper would have been impossible.

In presenting the summary of opinions I have received from my correspondents, I have deemed it advisable to do so, first by discussing the answers to each question separately, and second by giving the deductions that may be drawn from the answers.

In order to make a further estimate as to the influence of the kindergarten instruction on the mental and physical status of the child, other blank forms were addressed to first grade teachers and mothers who themselves had had children in the kindergarten. It is obvious that such a plan of investigation as I have followed is not without numerous limitations. It is not easy to frame questions that will elicit definite answers, nor is it easy to frame the answers in such a concise way as to convey in a few brief words the best of one's thought or experience; and it is clear from the very nature of things that the individual answer must have a fluctuating value. A partisan kindergartner, or a first-grade teacher who is a devotee to this form of teaching, will resent at once any implication that the kindergarten is anything but perfect. We learn, too, that the kindergarten conditions (perhaps this is no more true of kindergartens than other educational institutions) lack in uniformity. The differences in the institutions would explain in many cases the variety of answers received and would undoubtedly influence, to a large degree, the formation of opinions. Not only do the methods of instruction vary within wide limits, but, as one would expect, the teachers also vary greatly in ability and natural fitness. The children, too, are influenced by home conditions. The children of nervous parents, though coming from comfortable homes, present a problem somewhat different from children who come from uncomfortable quarters, where the advantages of culture and good example have been denied them.

PHYSICIANS' ANSWERS.

The physician is often consulted by parents as to whether a child should be sent to the kindergarten, and if so, at what age and what conditions would demand a discontinuance of attendance. He is appealed to for advice so often in connection with this subject that he naturally would have possessed himself of information which could be of value to his patients. The questions asked were mostly medical in character, but the replies received show that my correspondents had evidently given the subject much thought.

The first question asked was: "Do you commonly advise parents to send physically normal children to kindergarten?" The second question: "Are you opposed to sending physically normal children to kindergarten?" is so closely related to the first that the replies received to both questions may be considered together. Most of the replies were favorable; not a few were unfavorable and a few were indifferent; that is, the writer qualified his reply in such a manner that the answer was both favorable and unfavorable. So much depends on the child, the home environments and the kindergarten that kindergarten instruction may be valuable or harmful, depending on the provisions made. Therefore, these replies may be disregarded so far as drawing conclusions is concerned.

Those who are opposed to the kindergarten believe in the superior value of an outdoor life and unrestrained play; they deprecate the absence of ventilation in the kindergarten quarters, the complexity of the curriculum, too much play, the association of precocious, vicious and diseased children with normal children, the lack of competent teachers, the early age at which children are sent to the kindergarten, overstimulation and exhaustion of nerve centers and interference with the normal physical development, unnecessary exposure to infection, too much eye work. The following answers are characteristic of this group.

"I don't believe in kindergartens in cases where children have good homes; the best kindergartening may be obtained in the open air; there is too much eye work in the kindergarten and physical deformities such as scoliosis may develop."

Another correspondent writes: "Show me the child reared of sensible parents who look after the welfare of their offspring themselves, who treat their child as though it were a human being, confide in it, and it in turn, in them, who instill into that young mind seeds of common sense, self-dependence, righteousness, leaving out false modesty and deceit, who depend upon outdoor air, proper food and a quiet brain as a means of education, until this child is seven or eight years of age, old enough to attend the lowest class of the primary department of a decent school —show me such a child and I'll match him or her in health or disease against any conservatory raised, kindergarten, walked when-he-was-eight-months old, malnutritioned, myopic prodigy that ever drew the breath of life."

Another correspondent says: "I am opposed to the kindergarten because of the crowded schoolroom and the too early discipline and because the time should be spent in the open air. I think that the kindergarten is an abomination and born of a delusional belief that it is possible to make great men of little brains if begun immediately after birth."

Another physician expresses himself as opposed to the kindergarten because the normal child develops rapidly enough at home and does not need the extra or overstimulation of the kindergarten. Home training is better when done by a competent mother. There are, however, a few children of sluggish, semistupid condition to whom kindergarten work is of benefit, but for the majority it is harmful.

More than one physician referred to the fact that the teaching was not always what it should be, and that the teacher herself is often nervous or is too much impressed with a serious duty and is not simple and quiet with her pupils. In many of the replies from those who are unfavorable to the kindergarten, the position is taken that the responsibility of the mother is shifted to the kindergartner, and in a large number of cases the latter is an unsuitable substitute. Many physicians believe that the children learn nothing of importance at the kindergarten and that any attempt at early education of young children should be discouraged. As one correspondent says: "Babies ought not to be found in the kindergarten, but in the home." Or, as stated by another: "In good home training, the child gets the best instruction in a natural way without overstimulation. Kindergartens vary very much, but in my experience most of them have a very narrow point of view."

In contradistinction to these unfavorable opinions, several take a middle ground, as is expressed by the following:—

"So much depends upon the child, teacher, physical conditions in the school, and last, but by no means least, upon the mother, that it seems to me it would require close attention to many cases before any generalization should be attempted."

In the favorable answers, there is again brought forcibly to our attention the fact that three factors must be considered—the child, the home and the teacher. The correspondents agree that the points in favor of the kindergarten are that it teaches the child to observe in a logical, profitable way, it inculcates habits of discipline and obedience, observation, thought; it imparts a training that cannot be received at home, as a rule affords opportunity of social contact with children of like age, teaches self-control, makes the child democratic, independent, purposeful (especially in the case of backward children), gives them new ideas, makes them creative, encourages mental and physical development and is a logical link between the home and the school, which is in marked contrast to those who believe the kindergarten to be a haven or place of refuge for those children whose mothers are anxious to be freed of the care and worry of looking after them all day. Of course, it is presupposed that the methods of kindergarten instruction are carried out properly and that the child is given the training which the average American mother, with her nervous irritability, is not in a position to give. Excluding physical disabilities or congenital diseases, these correspondents are very much in favor of kindergarten instruction.

For instance, one correspondent summarizes his views as follows:—

"As systematic occupation for young children, the kindergarten fills a practical and decided need. When this purpose is frankly recognized and is not glorified into a cult and surrounded with mystic symbolism, there results a simple and useful combination of play and learning which appeals to children and gives them a better sense of rythmic and coöperative play than they get in smaller groups. It is only when the very simple purpose of this type of occupation is overlooked and the whole made subservient to principles and methods that rest on immature theories, that the kindergarten cult arises. This seems to me subject to abuse and to react unfavorably on children and teacher alike. Making due allowance for this form of exaggerated system-burdened procedure, and the equally crude insistence on a symbolism in occupations that carry their own interest and meaning with them, I cannot see that our use of this aid to early education has been particularly misguiding. The evil I call attention to has been generally recognized and the movement has come back from its period of exaggerated importance to a fairly well-defined and useful status in primary education."

Another correspondent says: "I have been an advocate of kindergarten training for many years, but I have been opposed to some of the abuses of the kindergarten, to its excessive symbolism, and to the preservation of some of the cruder forms in which Froebel expressed his principles. Better understanding of child nature, with the help of child psychology and physiology has improved much of the kindergarten material and kindergarten methods; but it has not touched the fundamental principles; in fact, the kindergarten idea, with its appreciation of the play instinct, of manual work and of objective and creative methods of teaching, is destined to pervade the curriculum of the entire elementary school."

Yet another correspondent expresses himself in this manner: "In brief, I might say that I believe in kindergartens for normal children, but that even here one should be careful not to push them very much mentally, and to watch particularly the effect on nervous children. Many of them are, I think, overstimulated by any kind of schooling. However, of all kinds of schooling, it seems to me the kindergarten is the best, since it attempts to make children think and observe rather than to crowd them with merely memorized data. With regard to children who are delicate physically, I think the matter is such an individual one that I hardly know how to answer it. One must balance the disadvantage of confinement with other children against the possible loneliness at home, and the absence of the association with children, which is often so beneficial. I am a decided believer in children associating early with others, in order to avoid the development of peculiarities which the petted 'only' child is likely to develop."

The next question asked was: "Should the so-called nervous children be sent to kindergarten?"

The opinions of the correspondents varied somewhat, some of them believing that the kindergarten often benefits some nervous children; others, that it is positively harmful, and still others taking the ground that if the kindergarten is under medical supervision it is of benefit to the nervous child, otherwise not.

It is desirable that these children should be kept occupied, and attendance at a kindergarten removes them for several hours a day from such home influence as may contribute to their nervous condition. Most nervous children stand in need of some kind of regulation away from home and friends. Of course, each individual case must be studied by itself, and if harm is being done the child should at once be removed from the kindergarten. By far the majority of the correspondents prefer not to send the nervous child to kindergarten. They say that there is too much competition; the child is under tension; the work is exciting; the restraint is injurious; the teachers do not understand the proper care of such children. On the other hand, those who are in favor of the kindergarten for these children believe that association with other children, discipline, occupation, training, direction of energies, are of benefit. One correspondent called attention to the fact that the so-called nervous child should not exist in the physician's mind and that analysis of the nervousness will reveal the inherent environmental vices, which are to be considered in the plans for the management of a nervous child.

Questions 5, 11 and 12 are so closely related that the answers may be considered together. They refer to the influence of the kindergarten on the physical development of the child; whether delicate children should be sent to kindergarten and whether the physical development of the child is retarded or improved by the kindergarten.

Some of the correspondents were of the opinion that the effect is a favorable one, because of the regular hours, systematic work and the influence of the teacher. Retarded children need special teachers, and, too, they are bad associates for other children. Outdoor life, unrestrained play, absence of overtraining, are important factors in regulating properly the growth of any child. Therefore, delicate children should be excluded from kindergarten, especially in winter when contagious diseases are prevalent. The kindergarten it would seem is valuable in physical development in most cases, and the sensible kindergartner will treat the pupils as individuals.

A very important question, in my opinion, is the following: "Have you in your practice encountered unfavorable effects on the nervous or mental states of children from kindergarten attendance?" While the correspondents gave many valuable opinions, I fear that in most instances they were based on isolated cases. Therefore, we find that they believe that nervousness is increased; that nervous children do not do well, being rendered more nervous and excitable; it makes them restless at night; they acquire habit spasm, and several have noted cases of chorea in nervous children as the result of kindergarten attendance. Very much depends upon the qualifications of the teacher to manage the nervous child. Headache, anemia, anorexia, downheartedness, low-spiritedness, hysteria, imitation chorea and an exaggerated self-consciousness are other conditions that were noted. A prominent New York neurologist believes that the kindergarten is a fairly useful institution when carefully conducted. He does not think that it does very much good or very much harm, and that one of its virtues is to give the mother a rest by taking the child from home.

The last question asked of physicians was, "Have you observed that children who attend kindergarten are more frequently, or at an earlier age, attacked by acute exanthematous or infectious diseases (including pneumonia and tuberculosis) than those who do not attend?"

One physician is of the opinion that there are more contagious diseases among the kindergarten children because their resistance is lowered by lack of physical exercise and fresh air. Others believe that the close association of so many young children, coming from all walks in life, tends to increase the danger of infection. On the other hand, a medical inspector does not consider the kindergarten a factor in the spread of contagious diseases; in fact, he says that any contagion would be more quickly recognized there than it would have been at home.

EDUCATORS.

The same blank forwarded to physicians was sent to prominent educators, but special questions on this blank were referred to them. Most of these correspondents believe in the value of the kindergarten, especially for the children of foreigners, and because it supplements home training and develops perception and imagination. The main thing, however, is the knowledge and good sense of the kindergartner. One man stated very emphatically that he considers the kindergarten the best educational feature of to-day. Another regards it as the best link between home and school, affecting favorably not only the physical development of the child, but also its mentality, making it less self-centred, less nervous, less likely to breed bad habits. Others say that the kindergarten opens the universe to the child in a systematic way and is productive of healthful development. Kindergarten instruction at home is good, but it is more likely to deprive the child of culture of association, which, on the whole, is valuable. It also makes better pupils in the grades because of the early training. Those who are opposed to the kindergarten believe that there is not enough freedom in it; that the children are kept in a constant state of tension and over-stimulation; the too frequent change of occupation; the young age at which children are sent to it. On the other hand, says one correspondent, a thoroughly good kindergarten, which really carries out Froebel's ideas of self-development and does not keep the child in such a high state of tension and constant occupation that he wants to be entertained all the rest of his waking hours, is most excellent training for school work.

As to the age at which children should be sent to kindergarten, the majority of those who answered this question qualify their answers with so many restrictions and provisions as to make it evident that the question cannot be answered positively, either yes or no. It is apparent that the degree of nervousness of the child, the regulation of the kindergarten, and the ability of the teacher to handle children will determine at what age kindergarten instruction should be begun.

As to the effect of the kindergarten on the physical development of the child, these correspondents nearly all subscribe to its value. It tends to develop the child, and only in very rare instances has it an opposite effect.

KINDERGARTEN TEACHERS.

Eleven questions were asked of each of the kindergarten teachers to whom the blanks were sent. The correspondents were selected with care, so that the answers received naturally would carry weight in coming to the formulation of conclusions.

Question 1. What proportion of children constituting your annual roster of pupils remain in your classes throughout the year?

The majority of these correspondents find that about two-thirds of the class remains in attendance throughout the year. Only one teacher gave a figure as low as one-half, and two gave figures as high as 90 per cent. The main reasons for a falling off in attendance are those caused by inclement weather or the fact that the children of well-to-do people leave the city during the severe winter months, spending them in warmer climates. It is very evident that the civic status of the child has much to do with attendance at the kindergarten.

There does not appear to be anything connected with the kindergarten itself, its work or its administration, which is operative in reducing the attendance.

Question 2. If there is an actual falling off in attendance, is it due to one of the following causes? (*a*) Contagious diseases; (*b*) nervousness; (*c*) failure of physical health; (*d*) acquired defects of sight, hearing or speech.

The nature of the answers to this question naturally would be dependent very largely on the relation existing between the teacher and the child's parents, because otherwise the reason for non-attendance would be unknown. Furthermore, kindergarten teachers, as a rule, easily lose track of the children because attendance on the kindergarten is voluntary. The child may drop out of the work altogether, the cause for this being unknown. The answers received to (*a*) show that contagious diseases are by far the most frequent cause for absence, particularly during those months of the year when these diseases are most prevalent. Nervousness, on the other hand, does not appear to be a considerable factor, and then only in the case of children who naturally are nervous or whose home life predisposes to nervousness. But what is of great importance in this connection is the fact that the work of the kindergarten, in the minds of my correspondents, does not tend to cause nervousness in healthy children. The same is true of (*c*)— failure of physical health—as a cause of absence. None of the correspondents noted any defects of sight, speech or hearing, although the answers to this question might have been somewhat different if these children were given the benefit of a medical examination. '

Question 3. What, from your experience, would you consider to be the most eligible age for entrance to the kindergarten?

Many of the correspondents are in favor of four years as being the most eligible age for entrance. Only one teacher thinks that six years is the proper age, and those favoring ages from three to four years are very few in number. The answers to this question show that from four to five years is the selective age when the child should be sent to the kindergarten. Some of the correspondents pointed out very aptly some of the features that enter into a discussion of this question, such as the number of teachers in the school, the physical condition of the child and its social environment. Some children had better be removed from home influences as soon as possible because of their pernicious effect on the mentality of the child, and some children are precocious so that they can enter the kindergarten at an early age. However, in the case of the normal child of good parentage, living in good surroundings, four years appears to be the earliest age at which kindergarten work should be begun.

Question 4. Has it been your experience that certain methods or particular kinds of applied kindergarten instruction produce (*a*) nervousness, restlessness or irritability; (*b*) disturbances of sight; (*c*) apparent loss of weight; (*d*) pallor; (*e*) bodily fatigue, and (*f*) decline in general health?

The answers to this question tend to show that kindergarten work does not produce the conditions named unless the work is too fine, such as sewing and delicate weaving, the instruction periods too long, the surroundings unhygienic, and the teacher too exacting; these conditions are operative not only in the kindergarten, but elsewhere, in the higher schools.

Question 5. Is the kindergarten more adapted to the needs of the children of the poor than to the children of the wealthy?

The majority of the answers to this question were in the negative, the correspondents being of the opinion that the kindergarten is equally well adapted to the needs of both the children of the poor and of the wealthy. One correspondent stated the matter very aptly when she said, "Both classes need the principles for which the kindergarten stands; but since the children of the poor receive less in the way of such an education at home than do the children of the wealthy, they naturally gain a richer experience." The principles on which the kindergarten is based apply to all, and cannot fail to profit all. Its teachings are beneficial to all children when efficiently and intelligently carried out.

Question 6. From your experience as a teacher, can you suggest any class of children to whom the kindergarten is positively harmful?

Unless the child is excessively nervous, or mentally defective, no harmful effect is caused by kindergarten work. All the correspondents were agreed on this, as might be expected.

Question 7.   Can you suggest any particular class of children to whom the kindergarten is of unusual value?

It must be apparent to all that certain classes of children would be benefited more by this work than others, and while a few kindergartners are of the opinion that all children are equally benefited, the majority of them believe that benefit accrues particularly to the only child, the restless, capricious child, the neglected child of the rich, selfish children and those lacking proper care at home; backward, shy children; children who are slightly deficient mentally, but not enough to be prohibited from engaging in the kindergarten exercises, and especially the children of foreigners.

Question 8.   Can you point out any kindergarten methods which are in general use or practice in isolated cases that you consider directly harmful?

The answers to this question proved conclusively that there are good and bad kindergartens; that the good ones are potent factors for good and that the bad ones ought to be abolished—the sooner, the better.   Baneful influences are very fine handwork; long periods devoted to such work; too many subjects in the curriculum; too much specialization; too many teachers; too much "showing off" of the children at exercises for the benefit of visitors; too many normal school students observing the children at one time; too much hurry and bustle; too closely following a set programme, and too little play.   It was also pointed out by one correspondent (and I wish to emphasize her answer) that often the harmful effect of the kindergarten on a certain child is overlooked because the observer mistakes excitement for interest. Another correspondent stated that "there is not enough gardening, outdoor work and play in the curriculum; that the fine drill of every kind should be displaced by plays and quiet occupations, demanding large, free movements, such as building with large blocks, modelling in clay, drawing with large crayons on large boards or papers, and such other occupations as are suitable for children of from three to five years of age.   For the older children, more difficult tasks may be prescribed, such as making things from thin cardboard, or wood, or cloth; such as little wagons, boats, houses, shops and so forth.   It is all great fun, quiet, and demands manual work and a wholesome, because spontaneous, quality of attention."

Question 9.   From your own knowledge, are the schoolrooms

used for kindergarten purposes suitable, so far as lighting, heating and ventilation are concerned?

It is apparent that each teacher answered this question in accordance with the location of her particular kindergarten. Those who are housed in suitable quarters, answered "yes"; the others answered "no." That there is room for improvement in this direction, we all know, because unfortunately many kindergartens are placed in the basement where they are out of the way and because the authorities feel that it is far more important to house the older children in the school suitably than to look after the kindergartens, where the children are in attendance for only a few hours during the day. We must insist upon proper hygienic surroundings for these children, even though their hours are short, because it is here that an impress—a most undesirable one—may be made on the child's physical health, from which recovery is not only protracted but may be impossible.

Question 10. Is it your observation that kindergarten pupils are too closely confined indoors?

Nearly all the answers are in the negative, probably because of the same reasons referred to in the comment on Question 9, and there are comparatively few kindergartens in which the pupils are not given a recess and in which outdoor exercises and work are not a part of the curriculum.

Question 11. State briefly what, in your opinion, are the best reasons for sending children to kindergarten?

The correspondents consider the kindergarten the best preparation for the work of the primary grades, for inculcating habits of concentration and industry, attention, respect for laws and an appreciation of individual responsibility. It places the child in its normal relationship with other children, teaches co-operation, is an entrance into an ideal community and a good preparation for the life-work. The child needs the child; it needs to have the joy of companionship and the incentives which come from imitation and suggestion; it needs to learn to subordinate self.

FIRST GRADE TEACHERS.

The questions asked of the first grade teachers had reference to the comparative value of training; that is, whether the children who have had kindergarten instruction make better progress in the first grade than those who have not had such instruction;

which of these two classes are most amenable to discipline and whether the former are more delicate or more nervous than the latter.

The answers to these questions indicate that, on the whole, the first grade teacher is rather inclined to look with ill favor on the kindergarten, except that the majority of my correspondents agree that the child that has attended kindergarten makes better progress than does the one who has not. The discipline in the grade school is more rigid than that in the kindergarten, and often it is difficult for the child to place itself unreservedly under the sway of the changed conditions. The kindergarten discipline, it seems, does not, in most instances, demand such strict obedience as does the school discipline. A few of my correspondents were of the opinion that the kindergarten children are more nervous than others, and one teacher stated that she would rather have children who have not attended a kindergarten. Another said that while the kindergarten children are more disorderly at first, they soon fall into the routine of first grade work.

It seems almost impossible to make any deduction from the views which I have obtained from primary teachers. While some believe that the children are more nervous and less amenable to the discipline of the school, others believe the children are more alert and receptive, and all in all make better pupils. The same diversity of opinion which confronts one throughout the entire inquiry occurs in summarizing the views of the first grade teachers and it is evident that it is difficult to make generalizations.

A few answers are so significant in this connection that I reproduce them in great part. "The kindergarten renders them adaptable to first grade work; but there is a great deal of namby-pamby, mushy control in kindergartens, with the idea of allowing children to do as they please." "I consider that children as a class who have attended kindergarten are more ready for school work and can make better progress than those who have not. They have been taught to act quickly in obedience to suggestions from the teacher and in unity with others, one of the most important lessons to be conquered early in school life." "They have been started in a systematic training of ear, eye and hand, which is a foundation for all the purely mental work of the schoolroom, as well as the construction and manual training work. Added to this, they have songs and rythm work, which are not only of value in an artistic way, but tend to promote good habits in breathing and bodily movement. Some time ago, when kindergartens were in their infancy, the correspondent thought that on account of the freedom and the play-spirit encouraged, the children were not as amenable to discipline after they had attended a kindergarten as when they came straight from home. Now she feels this is entirely changed, the play-spirit is so entirely hidden behind a constant occupation, along lines of interest to the child, that the work is all play and the play is all work. It is her belief that children who have attended kindergarten are less delicate and nervous than those who remain at home up to the time of entering the first grade. Children love companionship and thrive under it; and as they must have occupation, the constant variety of their work keeps them from growing weary of it and restless under it. But much could be desired for all schoolrooms in better ventilation, much more fresh air and cleanliness." "The temperament of the child, the character of the kindergarten, the qualifications of the kindergarten teacher would tend largely to determine the answers."

The following question was asked of mothers:—

"Please state in a general way your impressions as to the merits or demerits of the kindergarten as you have observed them in your own child."

Naturally, most mothers would make careful inquiry before choosing a kindergarten for their children, so that the mother's opinion as to the value of kindergarten teaching is of considerable worth in arriving at conclusions on this subject. Strange to say, however, quite a few of the answers received from mothers were unfavorable to the kindergarten. Perhaps this is the result of an error in selection on the part of the mother, or the fault of the child, or perhaps the system is wrong. Some of the mothers are of the opinion that if the mother will look after her child, giving it the advantage of a mother's care and guidance, the kindergarten is superfluous. One mother stated that for the mother who simply cannot train and raise her own children, and does not know what to do for or with them, the kindergarten is a godsend, both for the mother and child. Another mother found that her child derived the greatest benefit from applying the best of kindergarten methods and training to every-day life, without imposing restrictions, or sapping or over-stimulating the energies in the kindergarten. Others objected to the poor ventilation, the size of the classes, exposure to contagion, loss of sunshine, the development of a craving for amusement, making parrots of children, robbing them of fresh air, over-stimulating them mentally, and teaching them to play in school rather than to study. In my opinion, the following answers the question best: "Very beneficial when the kindergarten is of the highest standard, conducted in a large, well-lighted and well-ventilated room, and in charge of a woman who has made a thorough study of child nature. Under above-mentioned conditions, my child has shown a tendency to grow more systematic, more independent, and less self-centred. Under no circumstances however would I send my children to kindergarten unless there was one fulfilling all of the above-mentioned conditions within walking distance of the home, for I found that one week's attendance at a kindergarten of the type so common in most neighborhoods was very wearing, tiring the child physically and mentally, so that at the end of the session he would be too tired to eat the noonday meal and too cross to enjoy the play which before he had entered into with vigor and interest."

The favorable answers are equally characteristic. These mothers found that the child is taught unselfishness, given more wholesome thought and employment, bringing out its individuality and making it light-hearted and independent. At the same time, the child is given a pleasant occupation and good companionship. Emphasis is placed on the necessity of a trained teacher and proper surroundings, the home being the place where the balancing of effects is done. One mother said she had heard that children from the kindergarten do not make good pupils and that they expect to be amused and do not do things for themselves. She thought that this probably was the result of poor teaching. Most of these mothers are very loud in their praises of the kindergarten because they have found that it does so much to develop their children, not only mentally but physically; nervous, timid and excitable children becoming robust and happy. They believe in the kindergarten as a method of training the senses, inculcating the habit of obedience, cultivating powers of observation and developing the ability to mingle with other children at a time of life when they are inclined to be shy and awkward. Although kindergarten teaching has its drawbacks, say the mothers, the advantages far outweigh them. The kindergarten cannot be a substitute for home training, but it is often a safe refuge for little ones whose parents are obliged to be absent from their homes a part of the day, and therefore are unable personally to direct the steps of the child rightly. The child learns to respect the rights of others, to think of himself in relation to others and to develop a sort of community spirit. On the whole, these mothers believe that the kindergarten is a good institution and that it should be supported.

To pronounce the final word on this complex mass of evidence, and to reconcile the various conflicting opinions is obviously impossible. The proponents of the kindergarten system will find nothing to decrease their enthusiasm and the opponents to the system will feel all the more justified in their opposition. Yet, I believe, certain non-partisan deductions are clearly indicated.

In order to approach the subject with a better understanding, one must recall the origin of the kindergarten. Planted and reared in a soil rich in abstract philosophy, mysticism and symbolism, it developed into a growth foreign to our modern day concepts; and as a matter of course, the original Froebelian system is not in accord with our more recent knowledge of the functions of the child's mind and our acceptance of the modern scientific child study methods. To this end, a process of gradual simplification and the abandonment of obsolete forms has been necessary, lest the real meaning to the teacher and the value to the child be lost. Granted that the kindergarten conforms with the accepted child-study methods, the consensus of authority would indicate that children in general are not harmed by attendance. They may, however, be sent before they are of the proper age, which, in my judgment, is five years. Poor and neglected children are obviously benefited by the kindergarten. On the other hand, such children as have good homes, sensible, placid mothers, willing to devote time and care to their training, do not require the kindergarten. It is a question whether the kindergarten is the best place for the nervous and sensitive child. I would rather incline to the belief that brain rest is conducive to healthy brain growth, though even so one must modify that belief when the mother is believed to be incompetent or the home conditions unsuitable.

We have all met with that class of children who are nervous because of hereditary and environmental vices, and who do poorly in the home and poorly in the kindergarten. Such children would properly belong in school sanatoria equipped with specially trained teachers and located in the forest remote from the disturbing influences of city and town. Such sanatoria are being established in many parts of Germany.

The danger of contagion at kindergarten is a real one. It is

my own experience, as it must be of everyone who comes in contact with children, that the kindergarten is a distributing point
for the acute exanthemata and diphtheria; perhaps no more so
than the primary grades, but certainly the infection within the
kindergarten occurs at an age in the child's life when infectious
diseases are least desirable.

A word may be said in passing with reference to the hygiene
of kindergarten rooms. Many of them are overcrowded and are
ill-adapted to the purpose; not a few are improperly heated and
ventilated, and judging from many complaints made by mothers,
some are untidy. In view of these facts, no issue can be taken
with those who believe that the child should be in the open air as
much as possible.

While it is true, as has been so frequently emphasized throughout the report, that the kindergarten offers opportunity for social
contact with children of like age and gives the child occupation,
yet many mothers comment on the fact that their children became
more restless and were more difficult to entertain at home after
kindergarten attendance. The little ones desired frequent change
of amusement and lacked initiative.

It is impossible, from the answers received, to decide whether
kindergarten children make better progress and are more amenable to discipline in the first grades. After mature consideration,
I have come to the conclusion that the usefulness of kindergarten
instruction does not lie in the fact that it increases mental activity,
and I am satisfied that a child gains no intellectual advantage
in later life because it has attended kindergarten—for the same
reason it suffers no disadvantage because it has not attended
kindergarten.

Briefly, the kindergarten training initiates the child into school
life through the medium of playful occupation, which initiation
would occur in another form later on in the curriculum. The
kindergarten has its place. It is not necessary to all children; it
is unsuitable for some.

Perhaps no more important, yet on the other hand more delicate topic can be considered than the qualifications of the teacher
herself. It is not sufficient to say that not every woman is fit to be
a kindergartner. It would be more correct to state that the fewest
are fit to be kindergartners. Many of the evils of the kindergarten
may be eliminated by a competent teacher. A capable kindergartner does not permit the children to be over-stimulated. She

recognizes the capacity of her charges. She does not allow them to become fatigued because she realizes the physical endurance of the individual and the class. She does not keep them indoors when they ought to be out-of-doors. And more than all else, she is not enslaved by the symbolism of gifts and obsolete methods. An efficient kindergartner will lead a child by simple play.

In the final analysis, we are forced to the conclusion, as indeed one cannot fail to have been throughout the discussion, that each child must be considered as an individual. In other words, the desirability of the kindergarten depends upon the state of health of the child, the qualifications of the teacher, the disposition and capacity of the mother, the environment of the home and the equipment of the kindergarten.

STATISTICAL SUMMARY OF ANSWERS RECEIVED.

1. Of 119 replies from physicians, 66, or 55.46 per cent., were, for reasons medical or otherwise, in favor of kindergartens; 25, or 21 per cent., were unfavorable; and 28, or 23.50 per cent., were indifferent. Of those who gave unfavorable answers, answers were given chiefly on medical grounds because of insufficient or improper medical care.

2. Of mothers, with 70 replies, 43 were favorable, or 61.42 per cent.; unfavorable, 11, or 15.71 per cent.; indifferent, 16, or 22.85 per cent. Those in favor assigned the good results to social, moral and esthetic effects chiefly, and those of adverse opinion are chiefly based on insufficient physical care and danger of contagion.

3. Of 43 replies from superintendents and principals, 32, or 74.41 per cent., were favorable; 5, or 11.64 per cent., were unfavorable, and 6, or 13.95 per cent., were indifferent.

4. Of kindergartners, with 26 replies, 25, or 96.15 per cent., were favorable, and 1, or 3.84 per cent., indifferent.

5. Of 21 replies from primary teachers, 14, or 66.66 per cent., were favorable; 3, or 13.33 per cent., unfavorable, and 4, or 19.03 per cent., were indifferent.

6. From the standpoint of physicians: 42 favorable and 15 unfavorable replies came from the East; 17 favorable and 6 unfavorable from the Middle West; 3 favorable from the West; 2 favorable from the North, and 1 each favorable and unfavorable from the South.

7. As to the hygienic condition of the kindergarten, 12 kindergartners write particularly of proper and improper conditions of schoolrooms, ventilation, etc.

8. The best average age to commence in the kindergarten is five years.

9. 47.90 per cent. of all physicians favor kindergarten both for the rich and for the poor.

10. Concerning too early entrance to kindergarten, 48 physicians, or 40.33 per cent. of the total, have declared that this evil exists.

11. 40.33 per cent. of physicians admit greater susceptibility to contagious disease during kindergarten attendance.

DISCUSSION.

DR. ROTCH.—I am very much interested in this subject and I think that in the future we may be able to do a great deal by the proper management of the kindergarten. We should ignore the chronologic age of the child. Children should not be classified by their chronologic age, but by their special development. There are children of four years of age who may go and others of five who should not, for they may only have the development of three and one-half or four years.

DR. NORTHRUP.—In this age, when we are all interested so much in infant mortality, it may be well to think also along the line of preserving the children that are a little older. I saw the other day a child of six who sent me a nicely written note. She must have begun kindergarten when three. When I first went to school I was eight. In the future I think we may take more interest in the question of preserving these children while growing up.

DR. CHURCHILL.—I think the opinion about the kindergarten among medical men and a great many mothers arises from an erroneous idea of the true object of the kindergarten. The well-regulated kindergarten merely tries to *steer* the mental development of the child. It seems to me a logical thing to try to steer the young brain along well-regulated paths and that is all the well conducted kindergarten attempts. Unfortunately, I suppose, there is about one kindergartner in a hundred who properly grasps the idea. The kindergartner should be a very highly paid teacher, so that a very high class of women would be attracted to the work. The weakness of the system arises largely from the poor way in which it is taught by incompetent teachers. One objection raised is the lack of outdoor life that the children get, especially in the short days of the year, but this may be obviated to a great extent by having the kindergarten in the afternoon.

You often hear the statement made that the mother is the best trainer of the child, but the mother is not a professional, and I should much prefer to put the child in the hands of a professional than of an amateur. The kindergarten also tends to rub off the rough edges.

I have in mind a certain school in Chicago where the element of competition is entirely eliminated; no prizes are given; no attempt made to introduce that element. On the contrary, the spirit of helpfulness is taught. Personally, I am a thorough believer in the kindergarten, and I think we should try to steer the mental development of the child at as early an age as possible.

DR. CHAPIN.—One point that Dr. Churchill has made is very important, namely, that teachers for these young children should be better paid and have a better status than they do. The whole thing is radically wrong in our public school system. The teachers are graded according to the size of the children they teach. The early age is the critical time and yet they have the less experienced teachers. Some years ago I inspected the public schools of the lower East Side of New York, and found that the youngest children had the worst of everything; the poorest desks, the poorest seats, the rooms poorly lighted, and the teachers were the youngest. They allowed sixty pupils to each teacher. That is contrary to all principles of pedagogy and psychology. As these teachers become experienced they are promoted and take charge of the larger pupils. Associations of this kind should bring to the attention of educators that this system is not right.

DR. KERLEY.—My idea of the question is that it rests entirely with the surroundings of the child in his home. If the child can have outdoor life and proper attention at home, that is by far the best place. On the other hand, there are classes of children in every city to which the kindergarten is a godsend; children who go from squalor and dirt and bad air to well-ventilated rooms to be taught how to play, the necessity for keeping themselves clean, and the rudiments of living.

RECURRING EMPYEMA.

BY FRANCIS HUBER, M.D.,
New York.

Recurring pleural empyema, according to Dr. J. H. Pryor, is a term "employed to describe a renewed involvement of the previously affected pleura, occurring at an indefinite time after recovery from the primary attack." In his comments upon the case reported (*New York Medical Journal*, December 21, 1907, page 1,165), Pryor says: "The fact that empyema may recur years after recovery has not received the attention it deserves. It seems to be a very rare affection."

Dr. Park, in a careful search of the surgical literature, found no mention of the subject in the text-books. He found the report of a case by Ayer and another eight years after recovery reported by West. It is claimed that secondary attacks are apt to assume the sacculated or localized form, because of the pathological changes following a preceding severe involvement of a large part of the pleura.

The symptoms may be obscure in some instances, as in the case reported by Pryor. In others, the bulging at the site of the original wound or the physical signs will direct attention at once to the nature of the trouble.

In the above-mentioned article, Pryor, in commenting upon the apparent rarity of the condition, says probably the report of 1 case will lead to the remembrance or discovery of others.

Roswell Park, in the same vein, writes: "Regarding the rarity of this condition, I cannot believe that it is so uncommon as a search through the *Index Medicus* would indicate. I believe there must be cases of this kind on record, which are not revealed as such by the title under which they have been published; nevertheless, the fact remains that several pages of both series of the *Index Medicus*, when carefully searched, failed to show more than two such titles."

In discussing the cases, Park speaks of the interesting and unusual features; and, regarding its pathology, is inclined to regard it as an instance parallel to what one may see in the bones, as far as septic and suppurative disease is concerned. He recalls the fact that bone abscesses subside and remain latent for a long time, even as long as twenty years, and then are excited into activity, and develop, as it were, afresh.

As to the cause of recurrent attacks, Pryor offers as a conjecture that microbe life remained latent in a pocket formed in the process of healing, and became active under unknown favorable conditions.

The report of Pryor's case has led me to look over my notes. In the cases which have come under my own observation, there was little or no difficulty in making the diagnosis and instituting the proper treatment.

The usual signs of an effusion were present, and in addition there was a more or less distinct bulging at the side of the original incision.

Barney R., about four and one-half years old, was operated upon for pyopneumothorax about seven years ago. In this case a pleural fistula, which appeared to have healed, undoubtedly gave rise to the recurrences which took place after two years and after eighteen months respectively. Recently, after an apparent recovery extending over two years, a slight elevation of temperature, pain in the old cicatrix, followed by a purulent discharge, points to a recurrence. He is still under observation.

Perry C., about three years old, operated upon and discharged cured, returned to the hospital about two and one-half years later, with a sinus which had appeared a short time previously. Several operations were done subsequently. Patient passed from under observation and ultimate result not known.

Rosie A., two years old, entered the hospital February 6, 1906. She had been ill for ten days. February 12th the affected side was incised and drained; the subsequent course was favorable. The patient discharged April 1st with wound healed, pulmonary expansion excellent. December 23d was again admitted with a return, about ten days previously, of her old troubles. At the site of the original incision a small abscess appeared, which was opened, allowing 3½ ounces of pus to escape. Two ribs united with a bony bridge were removed; the cavity packed with sterile gauze. Further progress uneventful. Patient discharged January 30, 1907, in excellent condition.

Male, two and one-half years. Rib resected October 9, 1906. Recovery in about six weeks. Nothing abnormal until February 21, 1907, when rather suddenly a bulging appeared at the site of the former operation. Full recovery after another operation.

A girl, operated upon when about three years old, and who, when discharged, several months later, appeared to have fully recovered, presented herself as an office patient when about fourteen years old, with a purulent pleural effusion; and marked bulging at the site of the old scar. The subsequent course is unknown, as patient simply came for an opinion.

Finally the case of Bennie A. is cited. Bennie A., twenty-one months old, admitted November 7, 1907, with this history: Five months before, he had been operated upon in another hospital. He appeared to have recovered in about two months. Three months later he was admitted in a very bad condition, with the left chest full of pus. He was first aspirated because of his precarious state, and three days later a thoracotomy was done.

In explanation of such recurring attacks, the writer cannot add anything new to the remarks, or comments, of Park and Pryor. It is often a difficult question to decide when to remove the drain after an operation for empyema. If taken out too early, a little pocket may remain in a quiescent state, the superficial stricture healing nicely. We can readily conceive that as long as the general health remains good no symptoms may arise and no disturbances follow, until some accident or lowered resistance causes the old process to light up. In this manner we may readily explain the recurrences within two or three months, or after apparent cure. In other instances, in addition to the thickening of the pleura, there are abundant adhesions and pockets; while the greater part of the cavity may be obliterated and become innocuous, small foci may subsequently, at longer or shorter intervals, cause a lighting up of the original process and thus lead to a so-called recurrence.

ABSCESS OF THE LUNG DUE TO WIRE NAIL TWO INCHES LONG IN RIGHT BRONCHUS.—OPERATION.—RECOVERY.

BY FRANCIS HUBER, M.D.

New York.

WITH SURGICAL COMMENTS BY DR. HENRY M. SILVER.

In the *Philadelphia Medical Journal,* May 3, 1902, the writer presented "A Case of Foreign Body in the Lung—Diagnosis Confirmed by Radiography." The case unfortunately terminated unfavorably. In the present instance the results were favorable, and as many points of interest were present it is considered desirable to place the details on record.

Isie B., two and one-half years old. Was admitted to the Children's Ward in Beth-Israel Hospital, September 21, 1906.

History of summer complaint during the entire summer of the preceding year. Six months ago had measles, followed by pneumonia, ill about six weeks. Four weeks ago had a second attack of pneumonia, from which he recovered in about a week's time. As to further points bearing upon his condition, it is claimed that he has not been well for the past six months. Was supposed to have had whooping cough months ago, coughed considerably, expectoration mucopurulent. At no time was any blood brought up. Occasionally he would vomit after a coughing spell. More or less temperature had been reported. Has lost flesh, appetite is capricious, sweats profusely at times. Dyspnea present and cyanosis is quite marked.

Since admission the most prominent symptoms have been a paroxysmal cough, particularly marked when he becomes excited or lies on the healthy side. Vomiting occurs now and then, generally after coughing spells. The temperature has been of a septic type, ranging between 99°F. and 103°F., attended by irregular sweating and prostration. Loss of flesh and strength has continued. The dyspnea is pronounced and cyanosis of mucous membrane exists. Sputum (negative for tubercle bacilli) was distinctly purulent with excess of polynuclear cells. Prior to admission to the hospital several exploratory punctures had been made by the physician in charge with unsatisfactory results—the diagnosis resting between an encysted or interlobar empyemia and abscess of the lung.

Examination of nose and mastoid negative. Teeth and gums in good condition. Tongue dry and slightly coated. Throat negative. Conjunctivæ negative, no glands enlarged at angle of jaw. Pupils react to light and accommodation.

Physical Examination.—Chest fairly well formed. Expansion limited on the right side. Heart not displaced. Anteriorly, marked dullness over upper lobe of the lung on the right side, increased fremitus above, bronchial voice and breathing approaching the cavernous type. Posteriorly above, decided dullness and bronchial breathing. Over rest of right lung are found diminished breathing, voice and fremitus, with dull percussion note. Left lung not involved.

DIAGNOSIS.—Abscess of lung involving upper and middle lobe.

October 2d. Radiograph taken, but interpretation was not satisfactory.

October 6th. Exploring syringe introduced posteriorly in seventh inter-space, revealed a few drops of pus.

October 7th. Resection of rib (8). Lung was explored in various directions, but we failed to locate the abscess.* Gauze drain introduced and usual dressing applied.

Progress, as far as wound is concerned, satisfactory. On this day, October 26th, the physical signs simulated extensive consolidation of upper and middle lobe, due to occlusion of the opening. In a few days, as the abscess gradually emptied, the usual signs of a cavity reappeared.

November 14th. Fluoroscopic examination revealed wire nail in trachea and right bronchus, beautifully shown on plate.

When the mother was closely questioned, she now remembered that eight months ago the little one, while playing with some nails, suddenly had a distinct and characteristic suffocative spell, which soon passed over. The subsequent symptoms have been detailed above.

---

* Exploratory puncture has been considered the crucial test, although authors differ widely as to its value and significance as a negative manifestation. Such was J. B. Murphy's teaching in 1898. Tuffier says exploratory puncture is permissible but often deceptive, and when negative the puncture is to be made many times. He has made two to twelve punctures in each case and yet failed to locate the cavity in 17 per cent. of the cases of gangrene, 17 per cent. of the abscesses and 33 per cent. of the bronchiectasis. He claims that the procedure is harmless when done at the time of operation. Foul gas in the syringe is just as positive as pus. A radiograph may materially aid us in locating the purulent process.

November 20th. Low tracheotomy and removal of nail by the writer. (Description by Dr. H. M. Silver.*)

From the time the trachea was opened the pus and escaping air had a decided fetid odor. Tube removed November 23d.

November 28th. Wound smaller and healing satisfactorily. Over right upper lobe anteriorly breathing of a cavernous type with many large and small moist râles. General condition greatly improved. Temperature coming down to normal.

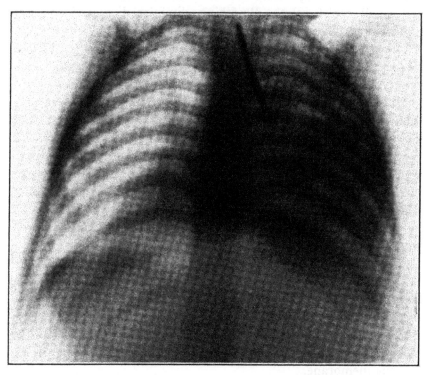

X-ray plate showing foreign body and condition of lung.

December 6th. Wound healed. Child is still troubled with paroxysmal cough, particularly when disturbed.

January 26, 1907. For the past seven days the temperature has been irregular, ranging from 98° to 103°, probably due to a mild infection from the pulmonary abscess.

February 20, 1907. Temperature had been normal for several weeks. To-day it rose to 101°F.; pulse, 128; respiration, 30. Following day temperature, 103°F. About this time a small abscess

* I would herewith gratefully acknowledge my obligations to my colleague for his valuable assistance and suggestions.

appeared at the site of the thoracotomy done October 7th. This was incised the following day and a small amount of pus escaped, revealing a small sinus leading to the pleura. Two ribs were resected to allow the chest wall to fall in and thus favor contraction of the pulmonary abscess.

March 17th. For the past three weeks temperature varied between normal and 103°F. Wound in chest wall gradually closing. General condition very much improved. Physical signs over upper portion of right lung anteriorly and posteriorly reveal large and small moist râles. Breathing diminished posteriorly, anteriorly somewhat bronchial in type.

June 9th. Progress favorable since last note. Sent to Willard Parker Hospital on account of severe nasal diphtheria and laryngeal symptoms.

July 1st. Returned to hospital in good condition. Temperature, 98°F.; pulse, 120; respiration, 30. Wound in chest wall discharging a little. Pulmonary signs about the same.

September 9th. For the past two months temperature normal, child doing nicely. Small sinus remains. To-day the temperature rose to 105°F., due to a slight involvement of left lung, which ran a favorable course in about five days.

September 17th. A small piece of bone discharged from wound.

September 29th. Wound entirely closed.

December 2, 1907. Since September 16th the temperature has been normal; great improvement in general health. Physical signs those of fibrosis of upper and middle lobe with dilated bronchi. The secondary result of the obstructed circulation is shown in the clubbing of the fingers and toes, with moderate cyanosis of the mucous membrane.

With a definite history and typical symptoms, little difficulty is met with in arriving at a diagnosis of a foreign body in the bronchi. The case is different when no such history is obtainable. In recent years the X-Ray has afforded valuable assistance, not only in establishing the presence, but also the location, of the body, provided it casts a shadow. The bronchoscope is the most recent addition to the appliances for examining the larynx, trachea and bronchi. With its aid the operator, in a large number of instances, is in a position to locate and remove the object accidentally inhaled.

In this part of the paper the principal and main features of interest center in the diagnosis. The history of a foreign body having been inhaled, was not developed until later on, the physical signs pointing to a more or less diffuse process in the upper and middle lobe of the right lung.

In general, in this class of cases, we are told that the child had been ailing for a longer or shorter period; the temperature is usually irregular in type, more or less dyspnea is present and

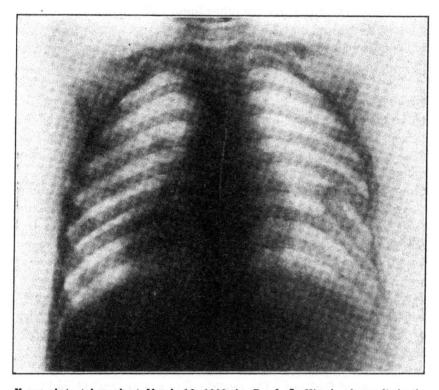

X-ray photo taken about March 16, 1908, by Dr. I. S. Hirsch, shows distinctly the characteristics of the chest walls from which several ribs were resected, and the changes in the lung. Compare with first radiograph.

cyanosis may or may not be found. Septic manifestations, as pallor, sweating, loss of appetite, diarrhea and emaciation are noted. Cough is common.

A very characteristic symptom, one which should arouse our suspicions at once, is ordinarily not interpreted correctly. I refer to the paroxysmal cough, during which the child grows red in the face and frequently vomits. The act is very distressing and is attended with a good deal of exhaustion. The spells are repeated at irregular periods, the child being comfortable in the interval. The attacks are more apt to occur during crying or excitement, and generally recur with greater frequency when the patient is placed on the healthy side. "The position assumed by the patient may effect the symptoms, especially if the body be movable. Naturally the position is assumed in which the foreign body is least disturbed." (*Modern Medicine*, Vol III., page 708.)

The severe coughing spells shift the body from place to place and even cause it to enter the other lung. This has occurred with a heavy object, such as a bullet. The paroxysms simulate whooping-cough very closely, now and then even the inspiratory whoop is observed.

The expectoration may be purulent, now and then it is streaked with blood. In a case under the writer's observation, the recurring hemorrhages ceased only when an iron nail was coughed out several years later. In some cases there is the characteristic odor of gangrene. The odor may be a prominent feature or may be noticed only during the paroxysmal coughing spell. Now and then, if our suspicion is aroused, a very careful inquiry regarding the onset of the illness may elicit the story of a sudden choking spell, attended by cyanosis, the patient appearing to be in imminent danger of suffocation. Such an attack may have been but of a few seconds duration or may have lasted for several minutes, but from this time on the "whooping-cough-like attacks" develop at irregular intervals. To bring out this point clearly and forcibly the following quotation taken from Carr's *Practice of Pediatrics* (page 681) is appended. "In some cases the presence of a foreign body is quite unsuspected, the child being brought some years after the accident on account of the expectoration of foul pus. On examination a unilateral fibroid lung with bronchiectasis is found, and by questioning the parents a history of whooping-cough at the onset may be elicited. This seems to agree well with the etiology of a simple fibrosis of the lung, and it may well be overlooked that the so-called 'whooping-cough' represented in reality the spasmodic attacks set up by the foreign body before it became impacted."

A. McPhedran writes: "The most difficult cases are those in which there is no history of the entrance of a foreign body. These cases often present the most anomalous symptoms. In all cases, especially children, with such unusual symptoms, more than half the difficulty may be overcome by bearing in mind the possibility of a foreign body. This cause should be present to the mind in all cases showing signs of local septic pneumonia, or gangrene of the lung, or of general pyemia with signs of early involvement of the lungs." (Osler's *Modern Medicine*, Vol. III., page 708.)

The prominent symptoms, then, are dyspnea, paroxysmal cough, septic temperature and possibly the expectoration of pus, or blood, or a fetid odor to the breath, particularly during the cough. Such a symptom complex points to a septic bronchopneumonia, localized abscess with or without gangrene, and, in the absence of other well-recognized causes, suggests a foreign body. To establish a positive diagnosis, an X-Ray examination must be resorted to. The method, however, is only of value when the object casts a shadow.

The physical examination reveals dullness, or even flatness, absence of respiratory murmur with diminution or loss of vocal fremitus and more or less restricted movement of the affected side. The signs are apt to vary in different cases and at different times in the same patient.

They will vary with the size and location of the pulmonary area involved, and the presence and absence of bronchial patency or communication. When a bronchus is occluded or the cavity is temporarily filled, the percussion will give a dull or flat note.

If, on the other hand, there is a direct opening, we may succeed in getting a cracked pot sound. Upon auscultation the sound will vary, depending upon the presence or absence of bronchial communication. In the former case, we may have bronchial, cavernous or amphoric breathing.

In general terms, in the overlooked cases, we have the usual evidences of a localized abscess with or without gangrene or the signs of a more or less complete consolidation of one or more lobes on the affected side, and, finally, if the infection is less virulent a chronic inflammation resulting in interstitial changes and possibly bronchiectasis, especially in cases in which there is only partial occlusion of the bronchus.

The diagnosis of abscess, with or without gangrene, or of a septic bronchopneumonia, etc., having been established, we must go a step further and look for the primary etiological factor. In the differential diagnosis the following pathological conditions must be considered: Localized empyema, an empyema discharging into a bronchus, interlobar empyema, pulmonary tuberculosis with rapid caseation, embolic processes from an old heart lesion, or secondary to a septic process in a distal vein, or chronic suppurating bone disease in the jaw, ear, etc., bronchiectasis, cysts (echinococcus or dermoid), and pneumonic changes due to pressure upon bronchi by enlarged glands, etc.

A careful consideration of the symptoms and progress of the case, with microscopic examination of the sputum and the use of the X-Ray, will materially assist in arriving at a correct diagnosis.

The diagnosis of pulmonary abscess having been established, the question of treatment arises, whether expectant and palliative or surgical. It is, of course, understood that the general condition must be improved by good food, fresh air and tonics. In view of the danger of tuberculous infection, the patient should be given guaiacol in regular and appropriate doses.

The surgical treatment will depend upon the size and location of the abscess and, furthermore, upon the presence or absence of pleural adhesions.

"Should there be an absence of adhesion and the lung collapse when the pleura is opened, and if the abscess communicates with a bronchus, it would seem from a theoretical standpoint that it should drain or close. Thoractomy in this manner is so easily performed that it appears to me applicable in the class of cases in which pneumotomy is most dangerous, *i.e.*, where there is an absence of adhesions. It allows of (1) drainage through the bronchus; (2) contraction of the cicatricial abscess wall; (3) peripneumonic compression from the air in the pleural cavity. All of these should favor the repair of the abscess." (J. B. Murphy's *Surgery of the Lung*, page 64.)

According to Tuffier 11 per cent. of abscesses of the lung are caused by foreign bodies. Now in the operative treatment of chronic purulent processes in the lung by pneumotomy, healing is slow and there is a possibility of a prolonged or permanent fistula remaining. In view of this danger the following suggestion of J. B. Murphy might be favorably considered.

"Abscesses without adhesions and with bronchial communications should not be treated by incision and drainage through the chest wall, but by producing collapse of the lung by injecting nitrogen gas or a liquid into the pleural cavity, thus compressing the lung and allowing the connective tissue in the wall of the abscess to contract and obliterate the cavity with the aid of the bronchial drain."

As the abscesses due to foreign bodies usually communicate

with a bronchus, the discussion of the treatment of other varieties is foreign to our subject.

Expectant Treatment.—In reviewing the literature, numerous cases are reported in which a successful result followed the waiting plan. The risks, however, are great, not only from the inherent danger due to the presence of the object, but from the secondary and later changes in the organ itself, with the subsequent possible development of tuberculosis.

NOTE.—Patient seen in October, 1908; general condition excellent, although fibrosis of lung still persists.

PART II.

SURGICAL COMMENTS.

BY HENRY MANN SILVER, M.D.,

New York.

Surgeon to Gouverneur and Beth Israel Hospitals; Consulting Surgeon to the New York Infirmary for Women and Children.

Since Professor Killian, of Freiberg, read his paper on bronchoscopy before the British Medical Association in 1902, the method of treating foreign bodies in the air passages has been completely changed. No longer are children turned upside down, slapped on the back to dislodge the foreign body, some cases even dying from spasm of the glottis during the procedure when surgical aid was not at hand. When the inversion method was not successful, the trachea was opened, tickled with feathers, or forceps, wires or hooks were introduced blindly in hopes to dislodge or extract the foreign body.

In order to make the diagnosis complete and the operation for removing the foreign body as simple as possible, every case should be examined with the fluoroscope as soon as possible, and a plate exposed. Do not depend too much on a negative fluoroscopic report—it is dangerously unreliable. Do not depend too much on a negative plate report, as cases are on record of pins in the bronchi showing no shadow until the fourth plate was made, others with two plates, as in our own case. Some non-metallic bodies do not cast a shadow, but they will cause a circumscribed shadow of inflamed tissue after they have been in a bronchus for some time. The advantages of an X-ray plate are the showing of the nature and position of the foreign body, thus enabling the surgeon to select a bronchoscope of the proper length. These advantages were very clearly demonstrated on the plate of our own case.

An operation for removal having been decided on, the little patient was placed on a table with a small pillow under his shoulder to make the neck more prominent, and chloroform very carefully administered. Dr. Huber made an incision an inch and a half long in the median line of the neck beginning at the upper margin of the sternum, dividing skin and superficial fascia; some superficial veins were clamped, divided and ligated, the deep fascia cut through on a director, the sterno-thyroid muscles separated and the trachea exposed. As the thymus gland appeared in the lower angle of the wound it was pushed down behind the sternum and held in place with a catgut suture. A needle armed with fine linen thread was carried through the trachea on each side of the median line and looped. Slight traction on the loops brought the trachea forward, which was then fixed above by a double tenaculum and three rings divided. When the trachea was opened large quantities of bloody pus escaped. When this was wiped away an endoscopic tube in the shape of a Burrage urethral and cervical speculum, 7 mm. in diameter, was introduced after the child had been placed in Rose's position. The endoscope was wiped out and a small electric light introduced. It was difficult to obtain a clear view of the bronchus on account of the pus welling up into the tube, but a dark spot surrounded with pus could be seen; this was grasped with a Noyes alligator forceps. When traction was made a sense of pressure was conveyed to the endoscope, which was withdrawn with the forceps. The foreign body, a wire nail two inches long, head downward, covered with black pus, was found to be in the grasp of the forceps. After the withdrawal of the nail, violent coughing spells caused more pus to be thrown out of the opening in the trachea. When the coughing became less violent a tracheal tube was introduced and the external wound diminished by one suture of silkworm gut below and two above the tube. The tube was removed in forty-eight hours and the patient's convalescence was uneventful. During the administration of the chloroform before the operation, it was noticed that the character of the respirations changed—they became labored—coarse tracheal râles were heard and the face was cyanosed. The anesthetic was immediately stopped and the head thrown forward; this diminished the cyanosis and difficulty of breathing, but did not remove the tracheal râles. A pulmonary abscess, ruptured early in the course of the anesthesia, without doubt, caused the above distressing symptoms, as was shown by the escape of a large quantity of pus when the trachea was opened. The experience gained from this case emphasizes the following:—

First.—Have everything ready before the anesthesia is started in order to be prepared to meet any emergency that may arise. This includes the presence of plenty of assistants and nurses.

Second.—Use chloroform as the anesthetic, as but a small quantity is required, and it does not cause a large flow of mucus. The chloroform should be administered with the greatest care by one skilled in its use, and it is well not to extend the head until the operation is about to begin, if the foreign body has been in the bronchus for any length of time. Jackson considers the "preliminary use of morphine, with its prolonged abolition of the cough reflex unsafe. The cough reflex is the watch-guard of the lungs, by which infective or deleterious materials are removed. The preliminary use of atropine to lessen secretion, as suggested by Ingals, is a good, safe procedure. It has the additional advantage of protecting the circulation from shock."

Third.—In addition to the ordinary instruments used to open the trachea, special instruments will be needed. The experience derived from our case leads me to put some form of an aspirating apparatus first on the list, for had it not been for the discovery of a dark spot in the pus, which proved to be the foreign body, it would have been very difficult with the means we had at hand to have removed such large quantities of pus from the trachea and bronchus sufficiently to have found the foreign body. Specialists and large hospitals can afford to have an apparatus operated with an electric pump. But a Dieulafoy or Tiemann's aspirator with suitable attachments, with an assistant to control the valves, or even a bulb-syringe can be used for this purpose. Cotton on holders can be used to remove small quantities of blood or mucus, or to apply adrenalin solution, 1-1000 if needed. Next, some form of bronchoscope will be needed, the use of the Burrage urethral and cervical speculum, together with the small electric light in our case, was perfectly satisfactory, because the foreign body was high up in the bronchus. In case of emergency, almost any endoscopic tube with a diameter of from 7 to 10 mm. can be used through an opening in the trachea. It is better, if possible, both in upper as well as in lower tracheobronchoscopy, to use Chevalier Jackson's modification of Killian's bronchoscope. The advantages of the Jackson instrument are illumination by a small cold lamp carried down to the extremity by a light carrier, thus doing away with the constant readjustment of a head lamp. The light being in the tube is always illuminating the object, regardless of the movements of the patient or operator. A small bubble or mass of secretion, or an instrument introduced into the tube, does not cut off any light, as the light is beyond. The tubes are also fitted with an auxiliary drainage canal, which maintains a dry, clean condition at the distal end of the tube. Both the lamp and drainage canal can be easily removed for cleansing. The operator should always take the precaution to have extra lamps on hand. The tubes should be perforated on the sides at lower end. When the foreign body is located, how can it best be removed? In our case the foreign body was easily removed with a Noyes alligator forceps. If it is situated low down in a bronchus, Coolidge's or Jackson's forceps are very useful. If it is an open safety pin, Mosher's or Jackson's safety pin closer can be used with advantage.

Fourth.—In young children giving a history of a foreign body lodged in the lower air passages for some time, it is much easier, in fact safer, to pass the bronchoscope through a low tracheotomy · wound. The opening in the trachea does not complicate or add to the danger of the operation.

PYELITIS TERMINATING IN SUPPURATIVE NE-
PHRITIS—CASE AND SPECIMENS.

BY J. PARK WEST, M.D.,
Bellaire, O.

The child from whom these kidneys were taken was a female ten months old when taken sick; her death occurred twenty-four days later. She had always been a healthy child, and had just been weaned on account of the mother's health. Her illness can be divided pretty definitely into three periods: the first represented by a lobar pneumonia, the second by pyelitis and the third by pyelonephritis.

I saw the child two days after the beginning of her sickness. A croupous pneumonia was suspected, but, owing to the late appearance of the physical signs, a positive diagnosis was not made until twenty-four hours before the crisis, which took place early in the morning of the sixth day of her sickness.

The second period of about ten days began on the evening of the day of the crisis by the temperature going up to 103° F., without symptoms on the part of any other organs. It is believed the pyelitis began at this time and was a direct result of the pneumonia. There was not now, nor had there been, any evidence of vulvovaginitis; it was only during the last period that a vulvovaginitis developed. While during the pneumonia the urine had been quite free, of a strong odor and stained the napkin deeply, it was now not so free, had but little odor and caused but little staining. On this first day of the second period, after three days' trial, a sample of one teaspoonful of highly acid albuminous urine was secured; it also contained a number of small cells and a few epithelial cells. The urine the next day was the color of milk and water, and for the next eight days was of a clean milky color. It was acid for the first few days; then became neutral, being slightly alkaline twice. The sp. gr. of but three specimens could be taken—it was 1014, 1012 and 1014. It always contained pus, albumen, pus cells in abundance, a great many epithelial cells of different kinds, and not a few blood cells. Altogether, about a half-dozen hyalin casts were seen. At times, the secretion was fairly free—at others scanty. On the second day of this period the temperature was 104⅜° and 104°, after which it went down gradually, until the eighth day it had almost subsided. There were never any marked excursions of the temperature, nor any chills or sweats.

For three days there was marked soreness over the entire body, and at all times there appeared to be soreness over the left kidney only. After the third day there was swelling of the face, hands and feet, which later extended up the arms and to the thighs, and pitted over the tibia. The child was very pale and depressed, but not wasted. At times she was very restless and at others took prolonged sleeps, and was usually dazed for some time after waking. During the first period she had vomited three or four times and the bowels were rather constipated; there was no vomiting during the second period, but on two or three days the bowels were loose. The urine gradually increased in amount and was usually passed more frequently, but was seldom free, and while the amount of albumen and pus diminished, they were never absent, and the milky color persisted. For three days now (thirteenth to fifteenth days) the general condition improved slightly and the temperature ranged from 99.4° to 100.2° F.

On the sixteenth day of her sickness, after three days of slight and gradual improvement, the third period began suddenly with severe gastrointestinal and uremic symptoms and continued until her death, eight days later. During this period there was never any fever and once the temperature was 98° F. per rectum. The vomiting was very severe and from twelve to twenty-four times in the twenty-four hours, while in the same time there were from four to twelve stools. Soon after the oncoming of these symptoms a vulvovaginitis developed. The urine was lessened again, although frequent small quantities were passed, excepting on two days (eighteenth and twentieth) it was fairly free. There was none passed for thirty hours before her death and about a half ounce was found in the bladder at the post mortem. The urine remained milky, but did not look so clean. There was less pus and a little more albumen. The cells—pus, blood and epithelial—were more numerous. An occasional hyalin and epithelial cast was seen, but infrequently. A sufficient quantity to get the sp. gr. was not secured. Every specimen tested for reaction was neutral. Most of these last eight days she was never fully conscious, and for two days (Wednesday and Thursday, or twentieth and twenty-first) she was semicomatose. On the third to the fifth days the right kidney could be easily felt through the anterior abdominal wall; after the fifth day it could no longer be felt. For the last three or four days she suffered so greatly that considerable doses of codeine had to be given her to control the screaming and restlessness.

The postmortem was limited to the abdomen. The pelvis of each kidney was thick and rough, and on the surface of each were a few small spots of distended capillaries. The left kidney weighed 80 grams and the right 72. This should be contrasted with 30.1 grams, the average weight for children of this age, as given by Bovaird and Nicoll in their tables in "The Weights of the Viscera in Infancy and Childhood" (ARCHIVES OF PEDIATRICS, September, 1906). Vierordt's table (quoted in the same paper) gives practically the same weight.

Dr. W. G. MacCallum, who kindly made the microscopical examination, sends the following report: "The section of the child's kidney shows a remarkable suppurative nephritis. The capsule is unaffected. The blood vessels are in general normal in appearance, although the smaller ones are distended with blood and there are occasional hemorrhages.

"Scattered through the tissues, sometimes in connection with disintegrated tubules, sometimes inside the tubules, there are clumps of bacteria. These do not appear to be in the blood vessels at all. They are bacilli somewhat larger than the typhoid bacillus. The tubules are very generally distended, with great quantities of leukocytes and desquamated cells. There are no definite abscesses, but relatively few of the tubules escape. The glomeruli wherever seen seem fairly well preserved. The remaining tubules show a most extreme fatty degeneration of the epithelium. The tubules of the medulla are uniformly filled with the débris of cells and leukocytes.

"The absence of glomerular changes and the presence of bacteria in the tubules and not in the blood vessels seems to argue in favor of an ascending, rather than a hematogenous, infection."

DISCUSSION.

ISAAC A. ABT, M.D., Chicago.—It would be well to cystoscope the bladder and learn something as to the nature of the bladder wall and also as to the orifices of the ureters, particularly in female children. The expert cystoscopist can occasionally throw important light upon these cases and render material aid, especially in cases where relief by operative procedure is contemplated but not clearly indicated.

A. JACOBI, M.D., New York.—Were gonococci found?

DR. WEST.—No examination was made for them. There was no history of former vulvovaginitis.

DR. JACOBI.—Undoubtedly the two belong together—the pyelitis and the vulvovaginitis. Was the uterus examined?

DR. WEST.—No.

DR. JACOBI.—It is a very common experience not to find a vulvovaginitis when it has existed for weeks and months perhaps. That is a result of the fact that the process is very frequently limited at that time to the uterus. The gonococci are stored away in the uterus. Up to the seventh to ninth year the mucous membrane of the uterus is not a smooth surface, but is in folds so that the gonococci may easily be buried in these folds and not come to the surface at all for weeks and months. That is the explanation of why we frequently think we have cured a case, when all at once it breaks out again—the gonococci could not be reached at all. There may be a gonococcal metritis a long time before it makes its appearance.

CHARLES G. KERLEY, M.D., New York.—Dr. West's case reminds me of one that I was called upon to autopsy. The child was supposed to have had malaria. There was a typical malaria chart, but autopsy showed extensive cystitis and multiple nephritic abscesses.

AN UNUSUAL TYPE OF ACUTE NEPHRITIS IN CHILDHOOD.

BY JOHN LOVETT MORSE, A.M., M.D.,

Assistant Professor of Pediatrics, Harvard Medical School; Assistant Physician at the Children's Hospital and at the Infants' Hospital; Visiting Physician at the Floating Hospital, Boston.

I have recently seen a number of cases of acute nephritis in childhood in which the characteristics of the urine have been materially different from those of the ordinary form, the chief differences being the complete, or almost complete, absence of blood and blood elements and the presence of a large number of small, round mononuclear cells, often associated with a considerable number of polynuclear leukocytes. There can be no doubt that these cases were acute and not chronic. The course was essentially the same as in other forms of acute nephritis, with the exceptions that the duration was usually shorter and the prognosis somewhat better. The following histories illustrate this type very well.

A boy, eleven years old, had had scarlet fever and measles when four, and diphtheria when four and one-half, years old without any complications. Since then he had been perfectly well, except for adenoids, which had been removed two years before. He went to the country about the first of August, 1907, and while there had no illness. August 17th he complained of a slight headache, and it was noticed that his eyelids and face were puffy. There were no other symptoms. He entered the Children's Hospital August 20th. The physical examination was negative, except for a little puffiness of the eyelids, which disappeared in forty-eight hours. There was no accentuation of the second aortic sound, and no enlargement of the left heart. The urine was yellow, acid, 1.030, and contained 0.2 per cent. of albumin. The sediment showed numerous short hyalin and fine granular casts, many leukocytes and a moderate number of small, round cells. The urine of the 26th was acid, 1.023, and contained no albumin. The sediment showed a few hyalin and fine granular casts, a moderate number of leukocytes and a few small, round cells. On the 29th albumin was still absent, but the sediment showed a few coarse, granular casts, a moderate number of leukocytes and a few round cells. He was discharged September 4th, having had no symptoms whatever, the urine then being perfectly normal. The urine has been examined a number of times since then and has been found normal. The boy has continued in good health. The quantity of urine, beginning August 24th, was 15, 22, 30, 30, 20, 26, 26 and 26 ounces.

This case is an example of the mildest type of the disease, with no blood or blood elements in the urine. It is impossible to say, of course, that blood may not have been present in the first few days, but as he was apparently seen on the third or fourth day, it seems very improbable.

In a number of cases which I have seen there has been a moderate amount of blood in the beginning, which has disappeared after a few days, the urine then taking on the characteristics already spoken of. The following case is an example. In it, however, the amount of blood was greater and it persisted longer than is usual.

A girl, eleven years old, had always been perfectly well, except for some pulmonary trouble for a few weeks when she was five years old. She was taken suddenly sick eight weeks previously with vomiting and slight edema of the face and feet. The urine was examined at once. It contained ⅛ per cent. of albumin and showed the characteristic sediment of acute nephritis. The blood elements disappeared very quickly, however, and did not return except for four or five days about a month from the onset. The urine increased from 1 to 3 or 4 pints daily. In spite of this, the edema recurred and free fluid appeared in the abdomen in the seventh week. The sediment showed no blood elements, but a good many hyalin, fine granular, coarse granular and epithelial casts of large diameter, and a very large number of small, round mononuclear cells with rarely a polynuclear leukocyte. The amount of urine diminished somewhat during the next few days, but the character did not change. Convulsions developed a few days after she was seen and were quickly followed by death.

The following case, which has been followed very carefully for the last two years and a half by the physician with whom I saw it in consultation, is a striking example of this condition. Blood and blood elements were present for a time in the urine, but always in very small amounts.

A girl, four and one-half years old, began to have a sore throat and coryza June 16, 1905. She had no fever, but one cervical gland was slightly enlarged. There were also a few enlarged

follicles on the posterior pharyngeal wall. The temperature continued normal. She was kept in bed as a precautionary measure
on the 17th and 18th. There was a little swelling of the legs on
the 22d, which was followed the next day by puffiness of the lids.
The swelling of the legs was more marked on the 24th. The
urine was then normal in color, acid, 1.026, and contained ½ per
cent. of albumin. The sediment showed many polynuclear leukocytes and a few small, round mononuclear cells. There were
numerous hyalin and fine granular casts of medium diameter,
and very rarely an abnormal blood corpuscle. Two days later
the urine contained 1 per cent. or more of albumin, and there
was rather more blood, both normal and abnormal. The urine
of July 7th contained 0.7 per cent. of albumin, many polynuclear leukocytes, an occasional small, round mononuclear
cell, many hyalin and fine granular casts of large diameter,
some of which were fatty, and very rarely an abnormal blood
corpuscle. August 4th the urine contained 1.2 per cent. of albumin. The sediment showed very many polynuclear leukocytes,
some in clumps, many large, round, dense cells, some caudate
cells and a few fatty, small, round mononuclear cells. There
were many hyalin and fine granular casts of large diameter,
some fatty and some with a few cells adherent. There was also
a moderate amount of abnormal blood. No blood was found in
the urine after September 1st, except during a period of two or
three days in late October. The urine a year later contained about
0.1 per cent. of albumin, a few polynuclear leukocytes, free and
in clumps, a few small, round mononuclear cells, and very rarely
a granular and hyalin cast, with occasionally a fatty cell adherent. The urine was absolutely normal March 6, 1907, and
has remained so since, except for a short time in May, 1907,
during an attack of whooping-cough, when it contained a very
slight trace of albumin and an occasional cast. The amount of
urine was somewhat diminished and the specific gravity high
during the first two months, after which it was passed in normal
amounts. The amount of albumin varied between 0.5 per cent.
and 1.5 per cent for some months, remained at about 0.5 per cent.
for a number of months, dropped to 0.1 per cent. in about a year,
and disappeared entirely in about twenty months. The most
striking things about this urine were the very small amount of
blood in a very acute condition, the large number of cells, both
polynuclear and, to a less extent, mononuclear, and the large

diameter of the casts. There was marked edema for a considerable period and, for a time in the beginning, ascites. The child has been perfectly well, both subjectively and objectively, for at least one and one-half years. She shows no signs of increased blood pressure. One cannot help feeling, however, that a chronic nephritis may eventually develop.

In some instances, not only is blood absent, but very few other renal elements are found, even when the symptoms are marked and there is a large amount of albumin. The following case is an example:—

A boy, twelve years old, who had always been unusually well and strong, had a moderately sore throat for a few days, beginning November 11th. The cervical lymph nodes were slightly enlarged, but there was no fever. He was not as well after that, got tired easily, and complained a little of shortness of breath on exertion. He complained of fullness in the head, had a slight diarrhea and nausea, and ran a temperature varying from normal to 101.5°F. for two or three days, beginning December 3d. The tonsils were slightly enlarged and reddened, and the enlargement of the lymph nodes persisted. He vomited December 7th and 8th. The urine on the 7th was high colored, 1.018, and very acid. It contained no sugar, but about 25 per cent. of albumin by bulk. The sediment showed a moderate number of granular casts and some polynuclear leukocytes, but no blood or blood elements. The amount was 1 quart. He complained of frontal headache and at times was slightly delirious, although he passed a reasonable amount of urine containing from 15 per cent. to 30 per cent. of albumin by bulk. He had several convulsions the morning of the 13th. Under treatment the amount of urine then quickly increased and the albumin diminished in quantity, disappearing entirely on the 22d. At no time were any blood or blood elements seen, while cells and casts were very infrequent. Now, a year later, his urine is perfectly normal and he is well in every way.

It is very evident from the examinations of the urine in these patients that the type of nephritis from which they suffered is different in many ways from the ordinary form. It differs from the usual form in that blood and blood elements are either absent or present in very small amounts, in the presence of large numbers of polynuclear leukocytes or small, round mononuclear cells, and in the comparatively large diameter of the casts. It does not differ in its symptomatology and course from the ordinary form of acute nephritis, unless it may be that on the average the cases are milder and the duration shorter. It may, however, as shown by these cases, eventuate in death, be accompanied by convulsions, or possibly develop into a chronic type.

I am entirely ignorant as to the pathology of this condition, never having had a case autopsied. The text-books say little about it, either because it is uncommon or because it is so common that it has not seemed worthy of mention. The only description which I have seen which seems to fit this type of case is one by Heubner. He describes in his text-book a type of acute nephritis "which is most common in diphtheria, but may occur secondary to other diseases, or even apparently primarily, in which the blood vessels are little, if at all, involved, and the cells of the tubules markedly degenerated. Hemorrhagic changes are extremely rare. The convoluted tubules are most involved, the descending limb of Henle's loop next. The urine is almost never bloody, the amount of albumin is moderate. The urine contains hyalin casts, casts with a little epithelium, renal epithelium and rarely leukocytes. The duration is usually short, varying from one and one-half to two weeks. There is seldom edema, more seldom uremia. Chronic nephritis develops even more rarely than in the ordinary acute type after scarlet fever."

This description does not quite fit these cases, however, because, although the urine did not contain blood, it did contain, as a rule, a large number of cells, either polynuclear or mononuclear, and the majority of the casts were of large diameter. It seems probable, therefore, that the pathological changes in these cases are somewhat different from those in the cases described by Heubner. Judging from the absence of blood, there is, in all probability, little or no change in the glomeruli, and, judging from the number of cells and from the large diameter of the casts, the pelvis of the kidney and the lower tubules are more involved than those higher up. In all probability, therefore, the condition is one of pyelonephritis rather than the ordinary acute glomerular or interstitial nephritis.

DISCUSSION.

Dr. Koplik.—Dr. Morse's paper calls to mind the description in Osler's symposium on typhoid of the kidney trouble, in which there are leukocytes and casts in the urine.   I have a case now under observation in which the existing nephritis probably resulted from gastroenteritis, and in which the urine shows small and large cells and casts.   The question in these cases is how to distinguish them from infectious nephritis with cystitis.   In these cases of gastroenteritis followed by nephritis, especially in young female children, there is a question of involvement of the ureters and bladder.

DR. KNOX.—One of the cases I shall speak of on Wednesday of urinary changes in gastrointestinal disease corresponds very closely with the description of Dr. Morse's cases.   There was hematuria, a number of leukocytes, a small amount of polymorphonuclear cells and a number of casts.   The case ran a very chronic course and came to autopsy.   Section of this child's kidneys showed the convoluted tubules undergoing hyaline degeneration, the nuclei not staining at all.   It seems that this belongs to this group of cases in which the degenerative changes are the most marked features.

DR. LA FÉTRA.—I had 1 case that corresponds quite closely with Dr. Morse's first case.   In my case the leukocytes persisted for a long time after disappearance of the casts.   I tried very hard to discover the origin of the condition, but was unable to find anything at all.   The child was otherwise in good health, and the only thing that called the mother's attention to the condition was some puffiness of the eyelids.

THE URINARY FINDINGS IN A SERIES OF INFANTS SUFFERING FROM INTESTINAL INFECTION.*

BY J. H. MASON KNOX, JR., M.D.,

Baltimore,

AND

J. C. MEAKINS, M.D.,

New York.

Concerning the condition of the kidneys in infants suffering from intestinal infection there has been a wide difference of opinion. In a careful review of the literature by Morse[1] in 1899 the conflicting views were graphically stated. Among those whose opinions are founded on large personal experience may be mentioned Kjellberg,[2] who in 1870 found nephritis on autopsy in 67 out of 143 infants dying of acute or chronic enteritis. In 3. non-fatal and 15 fatal cases of the same kind the urine contained albumin, casts and leukocytes. Holt, writing twenty years later in Keating's Cyclopedia,[3] asserts that, although cloudy swelling of the renal tubules is common in enteritis as in other febrile diseases, true nephritis is uncommon, and that albumin in large amount, renal epithelium, and casts are exceedingly rare. Nevertheless, Czerny and Moser[4] in 1894 found nephritis in 11 fatal cases of gastroenteritis in infants under two weeks old. The frequency of nephritis, they admit, diminishes with age. In the same year Falsenthal and Bernhard[5] reported a series of 15 autopsies in cases of vomiting and diarrhea in which the urinary findings had been repeatedly studied during life. Marked degeneration of the convoluted tubules was demonstrated. The collecting tubules contained many casts and often blood. In the urinary examination albumin was usually present and often necrotic cells, casts of various kinds and leukocytes were found.

Morse[1] presents a series of cases all in infants attending the out-patient department ill with uncomplicated diarrheal diseases in which the urine was collected by catheterization and carefully examined. The clinical diagnosis was fermental diarrhea in 64 instances and ileocolitis in 6. Albuminuria due to renal complication was noted in but 10 cases, 14 per cent., and, except in one instance, was of small amount. Casts were found in but 6 of these cases. No mention is made in this analysis of pus cells, although

---

* From the Laboratory of the Thomas Wilson Sanitarium.

in the table pus is recorded as present in the sediment in 4 instances, and in 8 other cases an occasional small cell is noted. No relation was made out between the urinary condition and any of the symptoms, and Morse concludes that the renal changes in the acute diarrheas are usually moderate in degree and degenerative, and not inflammatory in character. It is unfortunate that in each of the cases reported by Morse but a single examination of the urine was possible and that many of the cases passed at once out of observation.

In the same year Koplik[6] reported a series of 25 infants and children with acute or subacute gastroenteritis, in which albumin alone was found in 4 instances, albumin and casts in 13, albumin with casts and pus twice, and casts alone once, while the urine was normal in but 4 cases. Although Koplik thinks that these findings justify the term nephritis, he recognizes that the condition, on account of its rapid improvement without renal lesion, is different from the nephritis in adults or that after scarlet fever. It is brought about, he suggests, by the action of toxins in concentrated form upon the kidneys, because of the great loss of fluid.

Recently Chapin[7] found albumin in 75 out of 86 cases of disturbance of the gastrointestinal tract, in 37 of which casts were also noted. These elements were present in a somewhat larger ratio in a series of pulmonary and general diseases. The almost uniform presence of albumin, often with a few casts in many febrile affections in infancy, has been repeatedly noticed by Jacobi[8] and others. It seems, therefore, that although renal complications play a small rôle in gastroenteric affections of mild and moderate grade, yet in the severe forms they are more serious.

The present study was undertaken with the hope that a somewhat more extended analysis of the urinary findings in a series of infants suffering from diarrheal affections, and under constant observation in hospital wards, might indicate more clearly the extent and frequency of renal complications in intestinal diseases.

INTRODUCTORY STATEMENT.

The cases studied were those of 72 infants admitted to the wards of the Thomas Wilson Sanitarium.* They may be divided for our purposes into two groups—those with intestinal infection and those without. The urine was collected in specially ar-

* Hospital for children suffering from intestinal disorders, situated in the country ten miles from Baltimore.

ranged flasks or test tubes, or, in the case of girls, directly in a vessel or obtained by catheterization. In many instances a number of specimens were obtained from the same case.

The first group, the diarrheal cases, consisted of 53 infants; of these 33 had dyspeptic or fundamental diarrhea of varying degrees of severity, and 20 ileocolitis, as determined chiefly by the character of the discharges. In many of the latter cases there was evidence of intestinal ulceration.

GENERAL CHARACTER OF THE URINE.

In 31 of these 53 cases no pathologic elements were found in the urine; in 22 instances the urine contained albumin, casts, pus, red blood corpuscles, or several of these elements together, as will be specifically stated later on.

AGE PERIOD.

The infants studied fell into the following age periods:—

Birth to 3 months	5
4 " 6 "	14
7 " 9 "	17
10 " 12 "	5
13 " 24 "	12

Thus more than half were in the middle half of the first year.

SEX.

But little interest attaches in this preliminary analysis to the sex of the cases studied. They were: Boys, 34; girls, 19. Total, 53.

DURATION OF ILLNESS.

The duration of illness at time of urinary examination may be briefly stated as follows in periods of weeks:—

1 week or less	8
1 to 2 weeks	8
2 " 3 "	12
3 " 4 "	7
4 " 6 '	12
6 " 8 "	2
3 months	3
Uncertain	1

—

53

As the urine was usually examined shortly after admission, this date indicates that the babies when received were suffering from more than light transitory intestinal derangement. This is also shown by the result of treatment.

RESULT OF TREATMENT.

Discharged well..........	30......	57 per cent.		
" improved......	11......	20 " "		
" unimproved....	4......	8 " "		
Died	8......	15 "		

53

This table indicates that the cases studied were of somewhat severer character than those of the sanitarium as a whole.

Passing from the more general consideration to a study of the cases in which the urine was abnormal, a further analysis should consider the extent and nature of the urinary alterations and the renal changes, if any, indicated thereby. Twenty-two cases were found. It has long been known that in any febrile or toxic disease, a certain amount of albumin and some casts may be found in the urine, not because of an inflammatory lesion in the kidneys, but due rather to a parenchymatous degenerative process or "cloudy swelling" which the kidneys show in common with the other organs of the body and which may be of mere transitory character.

CLOUDY SWELLING.

Of the 22 cases, in 2 the presence of albumin was the only abnormality, while in 5 other albumin and hyalin casts were noted together. The albumin was never present in large amount, and the condition of the patients not particularly serious, with the exception of one infant who died of ileocolitis, in whom the renal condition was comparatively unimportant. All these patients had more or less fever; one had convulsions.

PYELITIS.

We regarded the presence of pus, polymorphonuclear leukocytes, in fairly large numbers in the urine as significant of a definite inflammatory process in the urinary tract. There was no evidence in the whole series of any urethritis or cystitis. The region of the bladder was repeatedly palpated in all our cases, and in no instance was any tenderness elicited. No frequency of micturition was noted. Pyuria alone or with moderate albuminuria without other change suggests pyelitis, although the exact extent of the renal involvement is difficult to determine. Cases belonging to this group were as follows: With pus alone, 2; with pus and albumin, 5, making 7 in all.

NEPHRITIS OR PYELONEPHRITIS.

When pus cells, together with albumin and casts, were found, the diagnosis of nephritis was made, especially when red blood cells or many bacteria were also present. This group of cases is as follows:—

Pus with albumin and casts........................ 4
Pus with albumin and casts and many bacteria....... 2
Pus with albumin and casts and red blood cells....... 2
                                                    ——
                                                    8

The casts were for the most part hyalin in character, though pus casts and granular casts were frequently found, but never in large numbers.

In regard to the character of the intestinal condition, these cases are divided as follows:—

Dyspeptic or fermental diarrhea................. 10
Ileocolitis 12

Dividing the cases with urinary changes into three groups, as above indicated: (*a*) albuminuria with or without casts; (*b*) pyelitis (pus cells without casts); (*c*) nephritis or pyelonephritis (pus cells with albumin and casts), the relation of each of these to the intestinal condition may be indicated thus:—

	Dyspeptic Diarrhea.	Ileocolitis.
Albuminuria	3	4
Pyelitis	3	4
Nephritis	4	4
	——	——
	10	12

This table suggests the conclusion that urinary findings may be altered by the toxins or fever in dyspeptic diarrhea, as well as during an ileocolitis. This may be because in many of these cases the two conditions are not to be sharply distinguished. A further analysis of the cases in respect to the intensity of the renal changes as indicated by the amount of albumin and the number of pus cells and casts shows about as severe involvement in the infants with dyspeptic diarrhea as in those with ileocolitis.

In respect, however, to the whole number of cases examined, the less frequent finding of urinary changes in dyspeptic diarrhea is brought out by the following table:—

	Total No. Cases.	Urinary Change. No. Cases.	Per cent.	Normal Findings. No. Cases.	Per cent.
Dyspeptic diarrhea......	33	10	30	23	70
Ileocolitis	20	12	60	8	40
	53	22		31	

An analysis of the cases with pathologic urine according to their age may be briefly indicated :—

Pathologic-Urine.

Age Period.	Total No.	No. Cases.	Per cent.
0 to 3 months..............	5	1	20
4 " 6 "	14	7	50
7 " 9 "	17	10	48
10 " 12 "	5	1	20
12 months.................	12	3	25
	53	22	

The number is too small to warrant sweeping deductions, but the figures suggest that urinary changes in intestinal disease are more frequent during the middle of the first year than at other times.

A larger number of our 22 cases occurred in boys than in girls; the number of boys in the series being 16, or 73 per cent., against 6 girls, or 27 per cent. This furnishes ground for the probability that the urinary changes were not brought about from without through urethral infection.

The results of treatment of the 22 cases with pathologic urine are instructive and may be indicated as follows:—

	No. Cases.	Per cent.
Well	9	41
Improved	7	32
Unimproved	2	9
Died	4	18
Total	22	100

The results of the remaining cases studied in which the urinary findings were normal were:—

	No. Cases.	Per cent.
Well	21	68
Improved	4	13
Unimproved.	2	6
Died	4	13
Total	31	100

Thus, as far as our experience goes, the general result of treatment of cases with normal urine was somewhat better than in those with altered urinary findings. Of the former group, 25 out of 31, or 80 per cent., were bettered, while 6, or 20 per cent., were unimproved, whereas in the latter group of 22 cases, but 16, or 73 per cent., were bettered, and 6, or 27 per cent., were unimproved.

The result of the treatment is also instructive in relation to the form of intestinal derangement.

CASES WITH ABNORMAL URINE. 22 IN NUMBER.

	No. Cases.	Bettered.	Not Bettered.
Dyspeptic diarrhea	9	9	0
Ileocolitis	13	7	6
Total	22	16	6

CASES WITH NORMAL URINE, 31 IN NUMBER.

	No. Cases.	Bettered.	Not Bettered.
Dyspeptic diarrhea	23	22	1
Ileocolitis	8	3	5
Total	31	25	6

Our tables must not be taken as indicating the effect of urinary complications in cases of ileocolitis. Of the 13 patients with ileocolitis having some alteration in the urine, 7 were bettered and 6, or 46 per cent., were unimproved, while of the 8 babies suffering with ileocolitis in which the urine was normal, but 3 were improved, and 5, or 62 per cent., were not bettered. In certain instances to be cited the persistence of urinary complications in ileocolitis are clearly seen. In several of the cases in which the urinary findings were negative, more frequent examination of the urine might have disclosed a pathologic condition.

CASES OF URINARY ABNORMALITIES WHICH DID NOT HINDER RECOVERY.

In many instances the abnormal condition shown by the urine did not seem materially to affect the outcome. Of the latter class 2 cases may be cited:—

CASE I.—F. S., Clin. No. 141, a child of four months, for the most part breast-fed; on admission had been ill for two weeks with vomiting and diarrhea. The stools were seven to eight a day and contained mucus and curds. There was no blood or pus in the discharge at any time. Repeated urinary examinations showed a small amount of albumin and a few hyalin casts with a considerable number of pus cells. The child vomited frequently on mother's milk. This was alternated with a low milk mixture to which sodium citrate was added. The stools quickly became normal in character, but remained five to six in twenty-four hours. The baby was discharged after three weeks apparently well, but with a trace of albumin and some pus cells still in the urine.

A somewhat similar case is the following:—

CASE II.—D. F., Clin. No. 229, a colored infant, aged eight months. About the history little was known, except that the child had been "boarded out," fed on condensed milk and table diet and for the past two weeks had had vomiting and diarrhea with eight to ten mucus stools a day. After admission the number of stools was considerably reduced, but they still contained mucus. Several days later albumin and considerable pus were found in the urine, but no casts. The temperature rose to 103°. The general condition of the child improved after this and the temperature became normal, but despite the liberal use of hexamethylenamin (urotropin) the pyuria persisted and was present on discharge, although the patient otherwise seemed well.

THE URINARY COMPLICATION AS THE CHIEF AILMENT.

In the next case the urinary condition probably indicated the chief ailment.

CASE III.—V. B., Clin. No. 82, a child aged one year, had had vomiting and diarrhea occasionally for a month. The stools never contained blood, but were largely mucus and numbered ten to twelve daily. The temperature during the whole period of observation, about seven weeks, showed marked daily variations similar to that in septic infections, sometimes reaching 105°F. Numerous râles were occasionally found in both lungs, but never any tubular breathing. Pyuria of a marked grade was present practically throughout. Only a small amount of albumin was discovered. Repeated cultures from the urine showed it to contain many colon bacilli. Variations in diet, irrigations and the persistent use of urotropin by mouth and rectum failed to affect the urinary condition. The child gradually lost weight, became peaked and emaciated, and died shortly after leaving the sanitarium.

NEPHRITIS AND PYELITIS.

In the two following cases of nephritis and pyelitis the urinary condition cleared up under observation.

CASE IV.—J. R., Clin. No. 107, a child of six months, admitted after an illness of about ten days in which the stools were frequent, mucus and occasionally blood-tinged. There was some elevation of temperature, and the signs of marked sepsis. The first examination of the urine showed a moderate amount of albumin, many hyalin casts, epithelial cells and many pus cells. Under a cereal diet, then one of diluted milk, and the use of hexamethylenamin, the condition of the urine gradually cleared and three weeks after admission was normal.

CASE V.—A. S., Clin. No. 175, a child of four months had been ill for three weeks with fever vomiting and frequent mucus stools. There was no history of blood. When first seen the patient was drowsy and the heart action irregular. The urine contained albumin and hyalin casts and a considerable quantity of pus. The temperature was irregular and ranged from 97° to 103°. On two occasions diacetic acid and acetone were present. Calomel and diet first of cereal and then of diluted skimmed milk, were given, after which the general condition improved, the stools became fecal and the urine normal.

In none of the cases cited—indeed in none of the whole series —were there localizing symptoms, nor was any pain elicited in palpation over the region of the bladder; there was no increased frequency in micturition, and no urethritis; in short, the leukocytes and other abnormal features of the urine could hardly have been introduced from the lower urinary tract.

SOURCE OF INFECTION.

The source of infection in these cases is apparently the intestinal tract, particularly the lower bowel. The infection reaches the kidney either through blood or lymph stream, or by direct contact. At autopsy one frequently finds a thickened and ulcerated colon lying immediately on a kidney. In repeated bacteriologic examinations in several cases in this and in other series, the colon bacillus, the predominant inhabitant of the lower bowel, has been present in the cloudy urine.

As has been stated, among the 53 infants having intestinal disease, 8 died, 7 of ileocolitis, and 1 of dyspeptic diarrhea. In 4 fatal cases, all of ileocolitis there were pathologic urinary findings. In the remaining patients who died, 3 of ileocolitis and 1 of dyspeptic diarrhea, the urine was normal.

CASES WITH AUTOPSIES.

Autopsies were performed in five instances: two in cases of ileocolitis with negative urinary findings, and three in cases also of ileocolitis, but with pathologic urine. A summary of the clinical histories of these cases with the autopsy findings is as follows:—

CASE I.—*Diagnosis.*—Ileocolitis (urine normal).

Patient.—I. S., aged seven months, Clin. No. 215, admitted acutely toxic and hard to arouse. The onset of the illness occurred three days before with violent vomiting and purging. The temperature was markedly remittent. The stools were mucopurulent, definitely blood-stained. There was some tenesmus. The urine was normal. The child, after a short period of apparent improvement, died from toxemia.

Autopsy.—On section, moderate cloudy swelling of the liver and kidneys were found. The mucosa of the large bowel from valve to rectum was thickened with considerable superficial loss of substance. The peritoneal lymph glands were enlarged. Microscopic examination of sections of the kidney showed considerable swelling of the cells of the convoluted tubules. The nuclei stained rather poorly. The glomeruli and straight tubules appeared normal.

CASE II.—*Diagnosis.*—Malnutrition, ileocolitis (urine normal).

Patient.—E. F., Clin. No. 245, an infant six months of age, weighing 9 pounds, was ill for a month with vomiting and diarrhea. Stools were watery, contained some mucus, but no blood. Under observation the child had no fever, but remained weak and listless and finally died of asthenia. The urine was negative.

Autopsy.—The heart was found to be somewhat enlarged and the mitral valve thickened. The mucosa of the lower ileum was swollen with numerous ulcerations of Peyer's patches in this region. The mesenteric and retroperitoneal lymph glands were hypertrophied. No abnormalities were noted in the other viscera. No section of the kidney was saved for microscopic study.

In the remaining fatal cases with autopsy the urine presented pathologic findings.

CASE III.—*Diagnosis.*—Septicemia, albuminuria, fatty degeneration of kidney and liver.

Patient.—B. R., Clin. No. 174, aged five months, was admitted with a history of vomiting and diarrhea of a week's duration. The stools were not frequent, but were said to contain mucus and blood. The child was drowsy when first seen. There was a large fluctuating mass in the scalp at the occipital region, apparently a suppurating hematoma. The mother proved indifferent, and real abuse of the patient was suspected. Albumin in moderate amount was present in the urine. The child had an irregular temperature and died, apparently from a general infection, four days after admission.

Autopsy.—Little alteration was found in the intestinal tract except for a slight increase in the lymphoid tissue of the large intestine. The mesenteric and retrosternal lymph glands were enlarged and softened. The organs, particularly the liver and kidneys, indicated fatty degeneration. The cortex of the kidney was pale yellow in color. The striations and glomeruli were not well defined. The renal pelves and the ureters were normal. On microscopic examination the sections of the kidney were found to stain poorly; there was marked parenchymatous and fatty degeneration, particularly in the cells of the cortical area, and but little small cell infiltration. The liver cells were largely displaced by fat droplets, particularly in the centre of the lobules.

In the above case the renal involvement and albuminuria were probably not due primarily to the intestinal condition, but to the general infection following the scalp lesion.

CASE IV.—*Diagnosis.*—Ileocolitis; nephritis.

Patient.—G. K., Clin. Nos. 246, 302. aged seven months, had been ill when first seen for two months with mucopurulent, frequently blood-stained stools. The child was markedly emaciated with scaphoid abdomen; otherwise the physical examination was negative. The urine contained albumin in considerable quantities, also hyalin and granular casts and pus cells. The patient was unusually lethargic, but seemed slowly improving when he was taken home against advice. He was returned a few days afterward much worse. The stools were all deeply blood-stained. He died in coma a few hours after his second admission.

Autopsy.—The absence of subcutaneous fat as well as the paleness of the musculature was a striking feature. There was marked chronic passive congestion of all the organs. The renal cortex was thickened and slightly granular. Several small uric acid calculi were present in the renal pelvis and ureters. The intestine showed the most pronounced changes; beginning midway in the ileum the mucosa was thickened and the seat of scattered punched-out ulcers increasing in number near the ileocecal valve. The large intestine to the rectum presented a swollen inflamed mucosa studded with numerous ulcers. The mucous membrane was in certain areas almost in shreds. The mesenteric glands were large and hyperemic. The urinary bladder was normal.

Microscopic Examination.—The sections of the kidney showed pronounced degenerative changes, limited largely to the cells of the convoluted tubules. In these the protoplasm stained poorly, was granular, and often contained numerous fat droplets. The nuclei were not stained with hematoxylin. In many instances the outlines of the cells were ragged and irregular. These changes were limited to the cells of the convoluted tubules. The glomeruli were little, if at all affected. The collecting tubules were normal. There was no accumulation of leukocytes or other evidence of inflammatory reaction

CASE V.—*Diagnosis.*—Ileocolitis, nephritis, pyelitis.

Patient.—E. B., Clin. No. 88, a baby of ten months, had been seriously ill with mucus and bloody discharges for a month. On admission the intestinal condition seemed improved and the stools but little blood-stained. The child, however, was pale and weak, and had extensive thrush in its mouth, and excoriated buttocks. The urine contained large quantities of pus and some albumin. There was some suppression of urine. The patient became progressively worse and died in four days after admission.

Autopsy.—There was found some fatty degeneration and congestion of the liver and kidneys. In the renal pelvis the mucosa was the seat of numerous hemorrhages; the congestion and ecchymosis extended down both ureters to the bladder. The lining of the small intestine was normal to just above the ileocecal valve, where the mucous membrane became markedly swollen and beefy with many ulcers, small and also confluent. The mucosa of the large intestine was congested and ragged throughout. The lymphoid structures were everywhere enlarged. From bladder and renal pelvis pure cultures of colon bacilli were isolated. The sections of the kidneys on microscopic examination showed marked degenerative changes in the cells of the convoluted tubules. These stained darkly in eosin-like amyloid material. The borders of the tubules extending into the lumen were irregular and many of the nuclei stained feebly. There was no evidence of acute infection and no increase in connective tissue.

In these last 2 cases the urinary condition probably arose from direct infection of the kidneys from the overlying diseased bowel. From the same source it is likely that constant reinfection occurred, and hence the pyuria persisted.

RESULT OF TREATMENT.

But little can be added from our experience to the treatment of cases in which there is abnormal urine. The nephritis as indicated by the amount of albumin and the number of casts is rarely of severe grade and tends to spontaneous improvement if the intestinal condition of the patient can be bettered. The diet was made as bland as possible, a cereal water was given with or without a small amount of egg albumin, and, as soon as it seemed safe, a milk mixture. In our hands a skimmed milk mixture was more easily borne than one containing more fat; although when the patient seemed able to digest fat it was given because of the desirability of reducing the proportion of proteid to fat and carbohydrate in the diet for a nephritic. When pyuria was the more prominent symptom, hexamethylenamin seemed of distinct value; of equal service were intestinal irrigations which emptied the lumen of the lower bowel of a certain amount of the infectious material.

THE URINE IN INFANTS HAVING NO INTESTINAL INFECTION.

For the purpose of comparison, the results of the examination of the urine in a number of cases which had no symptoms of intestinal infection are now indicated. These babies were suffering from the following ailments :—

Malnutrition	6
Diarrhea, simple........................	6
Intestinal indigestion....................	4
Congenital heart disease.................	1
Diphtheria	1
Marasmus	1
	—
Total 19	

In the urine of none of these was any abnormality found. An analysis of these cases as in reference to sex and age may be briefly stated as follows :—

Sex: Male, 13; female, 6. Total, 19.

Age period: 1 to 3 months, 2; 4 to 9 months, 9; 10 to 24 months, 5; 24 months and over, 3. Total, 19.

They differed from the infants already discussed in the fact that they gave no clinical evidence of gastrointestinal infection. As the nature of their disease suggests, they were not so acutely ill, although in some instances their ailments had been of long standing.

RESULTS IN THESE 19 CASES.

All were discharged well except 2, who died, 1 from congenital heart disease, and the other from marasmus.

To these cases may be added 1, the exact nature of which was somewhat obscure.

Patient.—E. S., Clin. Nos. 105, 220, a child of eighteen months, admitted with the history of having been ill for three months, in which time she had lost much weight. One week before admission there had been diarrhea, the stools containing mucus, "with some blood." On examination the child was found to be markedly emaciated with irregular heart action and respiration. The knee-jerks were much exaggerated and Kernig's sign was suggestive. The neck was slightly stiff and there was tonic contraction of hands and feet. There was evident mental impairment. The stools were normal after admission, and the patient improved on citrated milk. No lumbar puncture was made because of the rapid mending. The urine was found to contain a small amount of albumin, casts and some pus cells. The urinary findings persisted after the patient was discharged greatly improved. It was thought that this might have been a pseudomeningitis of intestinal origin, in which case the urinary condition was probably induced during the period when the mucus diarrhea was present. If so, the case belongs to the former group.

SUMMARY.

Urine of abnormal character was found in 22 out of 53 cases of intestinal infection in infancy.

Of these 22 cases the urine contained albumin and occasional hyaline casts as the only pathologic element in 7 instances, febrile or toxic albuminuria; in 7 others the presence of pus cells was the chief characteristic, pyuria (pyelitis); in the remaining 8 cases albumin casts and pus were all present, indicative of nephritis or pyelonephritis. The urinary changes were more frequent in ileocolitis than in dyspeptic or fermental diarrhea, though the extent of renal involvement seemed to depend less on the variety of the intestinal affection and more on its intensity. The pyuria persisted in some instances without apparently interfering with convalescence; in others it yielded to urotropin and in still others it developed into a serious and fatal complication. The infection seemed to have its origin in the intestinal canal from whence it reached the kidney either through the blood or lymph streams or by contiguity of structure. There was no evidence in our cases of involvement of urethra or bladder or ascending infection.

The autopsies made, though few, indicated clearly that, although the kidneys frequently escape injury during enteritis, they become the seat of extensive secondary changes in this as in other forms of infection.

The renal changes during intestinal disease in infants seemed to be those of degeneration, parenchymatous, hyalin and fatty of the convoluted tubules, rather than those of fecal infection.

In a series of ailments other than intestinal infections, and for the most part less acute in character, no urinary abnormalities were discovered.

REFERENCES.

1. Morse. The Renal Complications of the Acute Enteric Diseases of Infancy, ARCHIVES OF PEDIATRICS, 1899, Vol. XVI., p. 649.
2. Kjellberg. Jour. f. Kinderkr., 1870, Vol. LIV., p. 192.
3. Holt. Keating's Cyclopedia, 1890.
4. Czerny and Moser. Jahrb. f. Kinderh., 1894, new series, Vol. XXXVIII., p. 430.
5. Felsenthal and Bernhard. Arch. f. Kinderh., 1894, Vol. XVII., p. 222.
6. Koplik. New York Medical Record, 1899, Vol. LV., p. 451.
7. Chapin. ARCHIVES OF PEDIATRICS, 1906, Vol. XXIII., p. 329.
8. Jacobi. New York Medical Journal, 1888, Vol. XLVII., p. 225.

DISCUSSION.

DR. ABT.—It has occurred to me that these kidney lesions might be explained in the light of the work that has been done by Finkelstein on alimentary intoxications. If one would accept the explanation of Finkelstein that most of these intestinal disorders that we meet with do not depend on simple intestinal lesions, but are indications of perversion of metabolism with the production of toxic substances, much the same as certain constitutional diseases produce types of acidosis best illustrated in diabetes. This would seem especially true in view of the fact that the intestinal lesions are usually slight in comparison with the severity of the course of the disease. Following out this line of thought one may assume that the kidney lesions, so frequently met with in the gastrointestinal diseases of infants, are an expression of alimentary intoxication.

Lightning Source UK Ltd.
Milton Keynes UK
UKHW011026051118
331794UK00012B/1308/P

9 781528 401982